Just Tell Me What to Do

Start Living the Ketogenic Lifestyle to Lose Weight, Feel Great, and Reinvent Your Life for a New and Improved You

Kevin Davis, PA-C

ISBN: 978-1729031865

This book is dedicated to my wife, Dena', the perfect example of a Proverbs 31 wife and my best friend.

Contents

Now, discipline always seems painful rather than pleasant at the time, but later it yields the peaceful fruit of righteousness to those who have been trained by it.

—Hebrews 12:11

Chapter 1
Welcome to a New and Improved You

Just tell me what to do.

I hear this so many times, every day.

Why do I hear this?

I'm a longtime PA-C (certified physician assistant), and as of 2003 I've been running my own practice. Along with my staff I work with thousands of patients—and many of them are struggling with their weight as well as the health conditions that arise from being overweight.

What I see going on with them is that they try many different diet and exercise plans to lose weight. They try hard. But, when they don't find much progress after weeks of doing it, they give up. Understandably. And they feel frustrated. They feel frustrated and desperate for something that works.

Maybe you are experiencing the same frustration for the same reason: you aren't getting what you need to reach your weight and health goals. You've been trying with various eating plans, diets, and/or fitness routines, but you haven't made real progress. Most likely, this is not the first book about weight loss you have read. In general, every time you learn of a new diet plan, it leads you in many different directions— too many and too different. If you are here, it means that you haven't reached where you want to be—your ideal weight and ideal health.

Some of you may have many reasons for wanting to lose weight; others may have just a few. And you are all at different stages: perhaps you need to lose that last 10 frustrating pounds; or you are earlier in the journey and may need to lose 50, 100, or even 200 pounds. Probably most of you have tried different "diets" and have been influenced by the fads, the "diet of the year," but either you didn't get your desired results or have circled back to where you started. You stopped because either the foods weren't tolerable to continue for the rest of your life, or the plan was too difficult to maintain. I know, I have been there myself and have treated many who face the same hopes, frustrations, and failures.

From the Line to Quarterback

Going way back to my childhood, I was a chubby elementary kid. I didn't really care at that point that I was overweight. As I progressed throughout school, things began to change. In seventh grade, girls became more interesting. That new interest prompted me to make some changes (by the way, this is considered a *why*, which will be discussed in a later chapter—very important). In seventh grade, I played "on the line" in football. That's where they put the big kids. Over the next summer, motivated by my *why*, I came back weighing less after watching what I ate and after starting to exercise more. In the eighth grade, I was the quarterback, where they put the more athletic kids. Now, remember, that wasn't my goal, but it was a side benefit.

When I made changes in my diet at that time, I had no direction, nothing to go by except the "fads" that I heard about. Though I had a successful go at dieting at this early age, in the years since, I certainly struggled. The takeaway: I understand your frustration, and I am here to guide you, so you don't have to continue going through all the "diets" that I tried for years.

The most basic problem with the fad "diets" is the science. Most plans don't incorporate the findings from weight loss studies in a healthy, sustainable, and doable-for-the-regular-person way. We all have seen the boiled egg diet, the military diet, the grapefruit diet, but who can sustain such a disciplined and structured diet plan for the next 20, 30, or 50 years? I know I can't. We need to look at something that is reproducible, something that not just a few can do, but can be done by most everyone.

After years of trying out diets, probably trying the same ones that you have tried, I shifted gears. I started to look outside the box, at a different way of doing things. That's how I came upon the ketogenic diet and intermittent fasting, both of which we'll thoroughly explore in this book. As you'll soon learn, the ketogenic diet and intermittent fasting are based upon science—the actual physiology of the human body—(as opposed to a so-called health guru's wild food idea), and both are doable and sustainable for the long term. Yes, the ketogenic diet and intermittent fasting will entail you making some changes in your eating habits and doing something different. But, you'll be able to incorporate foods that you "have to have" while still reaching your goals. In adopting the ketogenic and intermittent fasting lifestyle, you won't be living a life of food misery!

Know that everything about the ketogenic diet and intermittent fasting that I offer in this book I do it all myself too. I have experienced results, great and long-lasting results. In starting the ketogenic lifestyle and doing intermittent fasting I lost over 20 pounds (which was my goal) and have sustained this goal for years now, and I feel great.

As a PA, when my patients come to me in frustration about weight loss, beseeching, "Kevin, just tell me what to do!" everything I'm offering you in this book is what I tell them. The result: hundreds of my patients have adopted the ketogenic diet and intermittent fasting lifestyle, and hundreds have lost weight and are enjoying better health. For example, take Clark H., one of my patients. With regular guidance from me, Clark started the ketogenic diet and intermittent fasting, and in less than 6 months, he lost over 25 pounds. Not only did his weight go down, his laboratory numbers concerning his cholesterol and blood sugar improved as well. Clark had to buy a new wardrobe—even new underwear! To this day, Clark has maintained his goal weight.

It's because of the success of Clark and hundreds of other patients that I'm writing this book. It will serve as your reference and guide. While everyone is different in their weight loss progress when they commit to the ketogenic and intermittent fasting lifestyle, all see results—with the long-term result of not only losing the weight, but keeping it off.

What This Book Delivers

Here's an overview of all you'll learn about in *Just Tell Me What to Do*. So you can get some helpful background knowledge, the next chapters delivers a brief history of eating trends and people's general health over the last 70 years. With this short history lesson, you'll get some needed context to better understand why the ketogenic diet and intermittent fasting are excellent and realistic options for regaining your overall optimal health in the long term.

After that, you'll find a chapter dedicated to your "why" and your health goals. In order to fully commit to the ketogenic and intermittent fasting lifestyle, you need to be very clear about why you want to lose weight and what specifically you want to achieve—so we'll address that.

From there, we move to the ketogenic diet. Over several chapters you'll learn all about the ketogenic diet, starting with what's happening inside the body when you eat—and how the ketogenic diet works so well by capitalizing on one of the body's very mechanisms for fueling itself—what's called "ketosis"—and in doing so, it ensures you burn body fat. You'll then learn the best foods for kicking ketosis into action, as well as how supplements and exercise can be incorporated into the lifestyle. After that—it's all about intermittent fasting—and please don't be worried! It's not that difficult! Next, we'll address any potential setbacks or stalls you might experience in the weight loss journey as well as common errors and misconceptions.

The book ends by reminding you of the baby steps to take—at your own pace—to get started into the ketogenic and intermittent fasting lifestyle. Also, you'll find a chapter dedicated to keto-friendly foods. It offers the core keto grocery list as well as easy recipes.

Wait—one more thing! At the end of every chapter you'll find personal statements and results from my patients, telling you about their experiences with the ketogenic lifestyle. These are key in motivating you

and showing you how you are a part of a greater ketogenic community. Additionally, if you go to www.ourketogeniclife.com, you can access more information about the ketogenic lifestyle as well as convene with other people in the ketogenic community to exchange ideas, offer support, and celebrate victories. Go to www.ourketogeniclife.com/book or to loveyournewyou.com/book and enter the promo code BOOK at checkout. You'll get to enjoy a discount into membership of this community. It's a special thank-you discount I'm offering to readers of my book.

I challenge you to consider your reading of *Just Tell Me What to Do* as an exciting journey where you'll be reinventing your life to become a new and improved you. That's how I experienced my education into keto and intermittent fasting—and it's how hundreds of my patients have experienced it too. Now it's your turn!

Simplicity: The Key

As I researched and read many articles to learn all I could about keto and intermittent fasting, one thing that kept coming back was to *keep it simple*. There is a lot of noise in the weight loss industry, and you can get confused about who to listen to. The one constant that is in my life has been my Lord Jesus Christ. Since He is the Creator, I thought, "Why wouldn't He have advice in this situation?" In 1 Corinthians 6:19–20, it says, "Do you not know that your bodies are temples of the Holy Spirit, who is in you, whom you have received from God? You are not your own; you were bought at a price. Therefore honor God with your bodies." That's how I see *Just Tell Me What to Do*. It's a book offering guidance on how we can honor our bodies, which is a means to honoring God.

This is what this book is about: helping you start a new lifestyle in a simple step-by-step fashion, progressing at your own speed—so that you can honor your body. We will go over everything, so you can start making the necessary changes. Following the steps outlined in this book will get you the results that you want.

If you want to go further, get even more information, and connect with others in the ketogenic community, please go to my website—www.ourketogeniclife.com. I developed this site, so my patients and readers all over the world—you!—can learn even more about keto and connect with one another as well. Please visit this website to find meal plans, grocery lists, and videos, which will help you to increase your understanding of the ketogenic lifestyle, so you can reach the goals you are aiming for.

As has been true for many of my patients, I hope that you take the next step and educate yourself about the ketogenic lifestyle and intermittent fasting—and ease your way into a new and improved you. Trust the process and look forward to the results that you desire.

Delana Stamper's Message

"Hi, my name is Delana Stamper, and I have been following the ketogenic diet since August 2017. I have lost 37 pounds so far. My health has improved, and I feel a whole lot better. I have energy that I have not had in years. I am exercising and walking every day. One thing about losing weight is that I get to buy a whole new wardrobe for summer. Nothing fits me that I wore last summer . . . Sure it takes a little will power and effort on your part, but in the end, it is worth it. There are a lot of foods that you can eat on this diet. I hope that this will help motivate someone out there that thinks they cannot lose weight."—April 2018

Blessed is the one who perseveres under trial because having stood the test, that person will receive the crown of life that the Lord has promised to those who love Him.

—James 1:12

Chapter 2
A Brief History of Our Health and Eating

Before we look ahead and see where we will be going, let's look back and see what we have been told in the past about healthy eating.

One hundred years ago, we didn't have the obesity problem that we have today. Sure, people probably worked harder on a daily basis—but I think more important than that is the type of foods that were available. Most people didn't eat processed foods, didn't drink sugary sodas and juices like we do today, and didn't have the convenience of the ready-made foods that we eat today. Most of their foods were natural—from fields that rotated crops and didn't use pesticides (which will be important when we discuss supplements later on)—and they didn't worry about eating the "fat" that is demonized today. They ate what they had: what they grew on their farm or bought at a local market.

When summer and fall came, they ate the fruits and vegetables that were in season at that time, not having the convenience that we have now with the local supermarkets. If you lived in the Arctic, the supply of fruits was very limited during the winter months. Having an apple wasn't even an option most of the time.

Even going back to biblical times, the diet consisted of proteins and higher fatty foods like olives and olive oils. No tropical fruits like oranges were available. Everyone got their nutrients through the foods that were available. God had a design. He made us, so that we didn't need to have carbs to live. We could get our energy from foods other than carbs and sugar.

1950s

Our current nutrition guidelines grew from recommendations that started in the 1950s. President Eisenhower had a heart attack. Due to his prominent position, doctors turned their attention to the cause. At that time, the cause was not known. Studies were lacking. However, a doctor named Ancel Keys had a thought. He thought that saturated fat was the cause, and he set out to prove his hypothesis. His study showed a correlation between saturated fat and heart disease. Thus, they cited saturated fat as the official cause for the president's heart attack. The problem was the study didn't show that it was a cause, but a correlation.

A correlation is a relationship between two factors. If it rains every time that you wear a blue shirt—that's a correlation. Your wearing that blue shirt does not cause it to rain. We need scientific proof of a cause-and-effect relationship, not a correlation. Dr. Keys's study did not show reproducible facts that saturated fat caused heart disease. No other factors were considered, and the subjects of the study were not random. If this study were done today, it probably wouldn't get published.

Numerous studies since then have tried to support Dr. Keys's hypothesis, but, to date, no study has been shown to say that saturated fat is a cause of heart disease. Much debate still exists in the medical community concerning the cause of heart disease. Ongoing studies are being done, and hopefully one day a definite answer will be found. But the one thing we know now is that more studies need to be done without any bias as to what the results will show.

1960s to the 1980s

Our culture began to change during this time period. Fast food was starting to take its roots. We started to look for convenience. Our lifestyles changed from a more laid-back style to a faster-paced approach. Dinners were now being prepared quickly and not from scratch, and the food industry noticed.

Then, in the 1970s, food began to change. More preservatives were added to our foods to help increase the shelf life and decrease waste. Also, more artificial sweeteners were discovered in laboratories. In 1897, saccharin was discovered accidentally by a researcher who tasted sweetness after researching coal tar derivatives. Then, in 1960 to 1980, cyclamate, aspartame, and sucralose came along. These artificial substances were then added to our foods. The underlying thought was that these artificial sweeteners were the answer to sugar consumption and offered the solution to the growing problem of weight gain. Plus, they were cheaper than sugar, and so the marketing began.

Following the addition of these substances, people began to gain weight. In response the weight loss industry came into existence, and even more new products were on their way to supermarket shelves. Over the years, these calorie-free substitutes have not solved our weight problems. We are finally now realizing that we cannot put artificial substances into our bodies and expect to live a long and healthy life.

The more that we tried to outsmart God's original design, the more we see that we need to go back to the basics. By eating foods that are more in the natural state, our bodies will feel and react better. It's taken several decades, but we are going back to the basics.

1990s

This is the period where we had more time and we wanted to become healthier. Gyms started to open, and new ideas popped up as the internet began to grow. New thoughts again began to appear while we hoped to find that magic pill or process to get the results we desired.

During this time, lifestyle recommendations were published. One such recommendation was to eat every 3 to 4 hours to keep the "metabolism" high. I have looked into this theory, but no studies have shown this practice to be effective. Also, I cannot seem to pinpoint where and how it originated. But just thinking broadly about the concept, it makes sense. The more frequently you eat, the more your body has to work to process the food. The more your body has to work, the more calories are used.

However, as with so many things, what we think isn't what is true. What we need to do is see what is backed by science, not just our thoughts. Sure, someone has had success with this plan as with almost any plan. However, if you are living a life that is hectic at times, this kind of grazing way of eating is difficult to manage. If I didn't have a job, children, and a million other things to do, I could probably do it. If I could just work out and spend another 3 to 4 hours prepping my foods, this plan might be a fit. As someone who did try this plan, this lifestyle is very hard to keep up. Always trying to plan a meal right after I ate kept me preoccupied with food. Having to have several meals a day became mentally draining. It was a lifestyle that I couldn't continue.

2000s

For so many years, we have looked at the models of calories-in-and-calories-out and eat-less-move-more. The thought was that if we could just control the balance sheet on this equation, then we should be able to lose or gain weight. Looking at the eat-less-move-more model, we see that moving more certainly can help. Nothing is wrong with exercise. Sure, we lose a few pounds and start to feel even better. The problem is, and I see this regularly at the gym, that if the diet doesn't change, then our exercise progress will eventually stall and our goals usually are not reached. We all have been there. We start to walk, lose a few pounds in the first few weeks, then nothing.

Then there's the calories-in-and-calories-out model. However, calories aren't the problem. All calories are not equal. If you look at a can of pop, the calories are clearly labeled on the front of the can. Why would they do this? What is the benefit? The food industry is trying to subliminally tell us that all we have to do is count calories. As long as we eat less than we need, we can lose weight. But we all know that 160 calories of a sugary drink is not the same as 160 calories of broccoli. The food industry isn't outright saying that consuming fewer calories will produce weight loss, but it   seems   to   be the implication. The marketing of the food industry accomplishes their purpose: sell products. The marketers are just doing their job, making a profit for the food companies. While there is nothing wrong with a profit, that's not my job: my job is to educate you so that you make decisions that benefit your health and make the decisions to get where you want to go.

So, let's look at an example. Say a person is eating 2,000 calories a day and their weight remains the same. That means they are burning 2,000 calories. The body wants to remain in homeostasis—staying at the same set point. We then tell that person to cut 500 calories a day, so they only eat 1,500. In the next few days to weeks, they see weight loss and get excited, but then it happens—the weight loss stalls. Why? Their body readjusts. Instead of burning 2,000 calories, their body lowers the set point and burns 1,500 calories. So then that person goes down to 1,200 calories. Again, they see some weight loss, but it happens again. Their body lowers the set point and weight loss stalls. So then here they are: they have decreased their calories but have not seen the desired weight loss.

When this happens to us, we get frustrated. We think, "Why am I doing this? I'm starving, and I'm not losing weight." So, we go back to eating 2,000 calories. Yet, we are still just burning 1,200 calories, so our weight goes right back up. The "yo-yo" diet. We all have been there. We all have felt the frustrations.

Today

Our grandmothers were right. Today, after all the studies and research, we are circling back to what was done years ago. People in the past didn't eat much sugar. Sure, we can improve some of the details and know more of the science, but the root problem really is sugar.

As we know now, sugar is added into many of the foods that we eat. Fat has been taken out, and sugar and artificial sugars have been added to replace what we thought was "bad." We have been programmed to think one way—fat-free—even though nothing has proven the fat-free route is the right way to go. We have eaten fat-free foods, but we seem to be getting fatter. Why is this? This doesn't seem to make sense. We were told that fat makes us fat.

A quote from the Harvard School of Public Health sums up a lot of the research being conducted now: "It's time to end the low-fat myth. For decades, a low-fat diet was touted as a way to lose weight and prevent or control heart disease and other chronic conditions, and food companies re-engineered products to be reduced-fat or fat-free, often compensating for differences in flavor and texture by increasing amounts of salt, sugar, or refined grains. However, as a nation, following a low-fat diet hasn't helped us control weight or become healthier."

But when they took out the fat, they added sugar. Why would the food industry want to add sugar? To make the foods taste better? Well, yes. To be able to produce more? Well, yes. To increase profits? Well, yes. To make us healthier? Well, no. Eating reduced-fat and fat-free products doesn't seem to be working. We know as a whole we are getting worse, not better. What's happening on the inside? How are these foods affecting our bodies?

One thing that we do know is that when these sugars are eaten, it stimulates many interactions inside the body that lead to detrimental results. The main thing that sugar does is that it activates the biological reactions that lead to unhealthy, frustrating results: higher insulin levels, higher inflammation, more heart disease, more diabetes, and more costs.

So, where does all of this leave us? What are we to think and how does this affect what we are to do? I'm guiding you through the process, as I have done with many in the past. In the next chapter, I guide you in determining your "why"—why it is you want to lose weight. You will also learn the importance of clearly articulating your health goals. The more knowledge you have—not just about the ketogenic lifestyle and intermittent fasting, but also about your specific weight loss and overall health goals—then the better equipped you will be to make the right decisions for yourself. Forget all that you have been taught before if your results haven't been successful. Give the ketogenic lifestyle and intermittent fasting a try, do what is recommended, and see what kind of results can be obtained in as little as 3 to 4 weeks. That's what you'll be learning over the course of this book.

Tina Caudill's Message

"Starting the next day helped me. It gave me the opportunity to research keto and come up with a meal plan for the following day. Seeing everyone's meals has helped me also. Seeing the pounds come off gives you an incentive to try again the next day and the next! Keeping track of the foods along with carb, fat, and protein content helped a lot. Even with being a nurse, I just never realized the carb contents of some foods I ate every day. Researching the carb content has been an eye-opener!"—April 2018

Every choice you make has an end result.

—Zig Ziglar

Chapter 3
Your Why

Clearly defining your purpose for wanting to lose weight is such an important but often overlooked step. Too often we do not take the time to figure out why we want to change. Having a purpose to put with a plan will help you when things get difficult and you want to quit.

Most likely, you have started different "diets" in the past, but something derailed your progress. You had a plan, but not a purpose. Do me a favor—try it my way. Your way hasn't given you the results you want. If what you have read so far makes sense, then don't stop. Let's keep on this path together.

Remember, "I can do all things through Him who strengthens me" (Proverbs 4:13). When times get tough, don't rely just on your own strength when there is a greater strength that you can rely on.

Your Why

Friedrich Nietzsche, a German philosopher, stated, "He who has a why can endure any how."

Every day I see patients who are struggling with doubt concerning their ability to lose weight, quit smoking, or make any big and important change. Typically, these patients tell me, "I try and I try, but I can't succeed at anything." To help them, this is what I say—"Imagine you had to come up with $5,000 in two months to buy a specific medication in order to save your child's life. Could you do it?" Their answer: yes.

Any parent would say yes to this and do whatever it takes to raise that money. They would work 2 or 3 jobs, sell what they had, and even ask others to give. No excuse would be given. Every avenue possible would be explored because the why was big enough to motivate them. This is where your mind needs to be in terms of making the changes to lose weight: your goal must be bigger than any excuse.

If I told you that by doing one thing you could almost double your chances of getting your results, would you do it? If you could increase your chances from 38% to 93%, would you do it? Then listen—take a few moments before you keep reading and consider *why* you are reading this book. What is your motivation? Why have you read this far into this book?

Determine your why now. Then write it down on an index card, and tape it to the mirror in your bathroom to remind yourself of your *why*. Look at it in the morning and the evening. Keep it on top of your mind. It's so easy to remind yourself of your why, but it's also so overlooked.

Goals

Start your process of setting goals in two time frames: in the short-term and the long-term. Set a short-term goal that will give you some motivation. This could be losing 5 pounds in the next 10 days, which is very doable following our plan. Having success as you progress will help keep you motivated.

Setting long-term goals will give you a vision. We all have an idea of where we want to be, the final result. For some, our long-term goal may take a few months, some longer. Having this vision will keep you in the right mindframe, not letting distractions take you away from what you ultimately want to accomplish.

Now let's turn to your goals—not mine, not your spouse's, not your parents', and not anyone else's. Just *your* goals. Again, don't overlook this part. Follow the process.

Your goals—write down all that you hope to achieve. These are personal. What motivates you is not necessarily what motivates me. There is no wrong answer, just your answer.

Be specific—don't say, "I want to lose weight." Instead, write down how much you want to lose. If that number is 10, 20, or even 50, that's OK. It is your goal. It may be that you want to fit into a certain dress. If so, write it down. Maybe your goal is to get off medication. If you are a diabetic, maybe there is a possibility that you can, or even at least decrease the dose. Just be specific on the dose.

Give it a timeframe—it's not, "I want to lose 10 pounds"; it is, "I want to lose 10 pounds in the next 6 weeks," or "I want to fit into those pants in 2 months." Once you give yourself a timeframe, it becomes more real.

State your how—how do you get to where you want to go? This is my website can give you additional help: www.ourketogeniclife.com. (Remember to use the discount code—BOOK at checkout at our website www.ourketoketogeniclife.com/book—that I'm offering exclusively to readers of this book!) At this site I've laid out the baby steps I use to help people start and maintain a new lifestyle. You'll find everything you need to start and how to do it; you just need to commit to yourself. We'll also be looking at similar information in this book. Remember, a journey starts with one step. You can't get to step 10 without starting at step one.

If you decide losing weight and regaining your health is something that is not so important to you, then it is more of a dream and not a goal. For example, I dream of having a 6-pack abs, but it is not currently a goal. We all would like to have those model-type abs, of course, but for most of us, the goal is being healthy, not getting on the cover of a magazine.

Zig Ziglar gave a profound analogy. He was asked at a conference if he was going to motivate the people attending and get them fired up. He said that of course he was going to try to do his best. They then asked him if that motivation was going to last or if it would fizzle out in a few days. His response was golden: "Motivation is like bathing. It's good to bathe today, but that bath isn't going to last forever. You have to get up each day and bathe again. I can help you with developing some tools to get up each day and refocus, to continue on a path to your goals. But you must put them into action, getting up each day and reminding yourself of where you want to go."

Accountability Partner

If we keep everything a secret, if our goals are known only to us, a funny thing happens. When we "talk" to ourselves, we tend to be more lenient on our progress than if we were evaluating someone else. We tend to judge ourselves by our intentions rather than our actual behaviors.

I know this is true for the patients I see in my clinic. If a person comes in frequently and together we closely track their progress, then that person does better. If they only come in every few months, the results lack. When they get off-track, they usually say something like: "I forgot to bring my lunch all last week, so I 'had' to go out with my co-workers and nothing was available that I should be eating. I 'meant' to bring my lunch. I had every good intention. It wasn't my fault."

Now if you had to report to someone, someone who wouldn't let you off with excuses, maybe your behavior would be different. The night before you are more likely to remember that you need to take some time to make a lunch, knowing that your "intention" can't be used as an excuse.

So before you start, think and tell someone what you are planning to do. Let them know you are getting ready to change your whole life, your daily decisions, and you want them to check in with you regularly to see how you are doing, to encourage you as you make changes, and to walk with you through this journey to start a *new you*!

Remember this one thing as you start—change requires change. You don't have to make every recommended change given in this book right at the start. But what you need to do is look to change your habits, little by little. You might choose to make all the changes in one go or just ease yourself into the plan, making a few changes at a time. You can be like the person who wants to just rip the Band-Aid off and jump full body in the pool, or you can ease that Band-Aid off and first put your toes in the water. Either way is OK, but the key is to commit, start, and do it today.

Your direction—your why and goals combined with your baby steps—will get you to your destiny. Remember, go to www.ourketogeniclife.com to find those baby steps. Empower yourself with the information offered on the site and the community members you'll find there too.

In the next chapter, we're going inside the human body to learn how the body gets fuel from food you eat. Once you understand this mechanism, you'll see how the ketogenic diet works to ensure you burn fat instead of storing it on your body!

Julia S.'s Statistics

Julia is a 74-year-old female who was on insulin (50 units) every night. On May 17, 2017, Julia's initial hemoglobin A1c was 10.3 with an average blood sugar of 280 (normal is less than 6.0 A1c with an average blood sugar of 136). After stopping her insulin and controlling her sugar by the ketogenic diet alone, her A1c dropped to 6.3 with an average blood sugar of 147. She has lost over 20 pounds and has developed a new lifestyle, a new *ketogenic* lifestyle.

Direction, not intention, determines your destination.

—Andy Stanley

Chapter 4
Hormones and *The* Hormone

Now some basic biology, so you can better understand what's going on in the body that affects weight loss.

Hormones are substances in your body that act as chemical messengers. Produced by glands, like the thyroid or adrenals, hormones travel to other parts of the body to signal and regulate the activity of the cells and organs. It gets very complicated because many things affect when hormones are produced and how much or how little is produced. Hormones can even affect each other.

Most of this is not really that necessary to know, but I want you to understand one important concept: what **mainly** controls your weight loss boils down to trying to affect these hormones in a positive way. We will either affect these hormones in a good or a bad way; we have a choice.

Insulin—The Key

As we started to discuss already, sugar plays a big role in weight loss. For so many years, we have looked at the wrong key factor: fat. However, we now know that it's our daily sugar intake that's plays the most important role in weight loss. What this means then— fat does not cause you to be fat. Sugar, in fact, is the culprit.

Your body needs an energy source. Although not the best, sugar is the quickest and easiest source for that. This molecule can be broken down and used very quickly. It isn't the most efficient, but it can be used to supply what your body needs.

The most effective source of energy is actually fat. Surprised? Many are. The problem is most of the time the body never gets to that source. As long as sugar is available, the body will use that as its source of energy, then store the excess as fat for future use.

So what does that have to do with hormones? What you are eating is affecting your entire body, not just your hunger. Remember that weight loss and getting healthy are not only about calories. Many interactions between food and your body are occurring every day, and hormones are involved in almost all these interactions.

There are many hormones that affect your weight and health. The hormone produced by the thyroid is probably the most common hormone people want checked. They think that if they have an underactive thyroid, correcting that will result in weight loss. While that may help, it usually doesn't get them the results they desire.

Many other hormones also affect our weight. Two hormones in your stomach affect your daily food intake. A hormone called leptin, AKA the satiety hormone, tells us when we are full. Another hormone called ghrelin, AKA the hunger hormone, tells us when we are hungry. This can all get confusing, and many of us aren't interested in the minutiae of how our bodies process all that we eat and how it affects our weight. So, we need to make things simple, so everyone can understand and follow. This is where I want you to start. The only hormone I want you to follow for now is the insulin hormone.

When we eat carbohydrates, the cells in our body want to use the sugar (glucose) from those carbohydrates for energy. However, the sugar needs to reach those cells. That's where insulin comes in. When we eat , the pancreas is stimulated and it produces more insulin. The insulin is responsible for taking sugar (glucose) and "unlocking" cells in the body, so they can use that sugar to make energy. This is the job of insulin: when a person eats carbohydrates, insulin is responsible for taking the sugar to cells, so they can use the sugar for energy.

Something else to know about insulin is its relationship to blood sugar or glucose. Because insulin works to regulate blood sugar levels as described in the previous paragraph, the two have a parallel relationship. What this means is that when a person eats carbohydrates and their blood sugar rises from the glucose from those carbohydrates, the result of that is their insulin levels also rises. When a person's blood sugar falls, their insulin level also drops.

Now that you know how insulin generally works in the body, I want you to focus your attention on this one aspect. I want you to concentrate on insulin's role in "fat storage." As far as we are concerned, those two terms are interchangeable. The more insulin you have, the more fat you store. The less insulin you have, the less fat you store. This is scientific, not my hypothesis. If I give you insulin, you will gain weight. If a mom brings to my clinic her child who eats just fine but isn't gaining weight, and we find they have insulin-dependent diabetes and start the child on insulin, then they will gain weight. So, you should be trying to control insulin.

If we are able to decrease the production of insulin, we should be able to lose weight. The lower the insulin, the greater the weight loss. This is what my staff, many of my patients, and I have been doing with the ketogenic diet and getting results in a constant, reproducible way.

When we eat, that food is going to affect us somehow. If we want to decrease insulin as the basis of our lifestyle, then you need to know which foods make it go up and which foods make it go down. Let's look at what the science tells us. After researching much of the literature, I have found two things we should concentrate on: 1—what we eat and 2—when we eat. This is the easiest and best way to start.

What We Eat

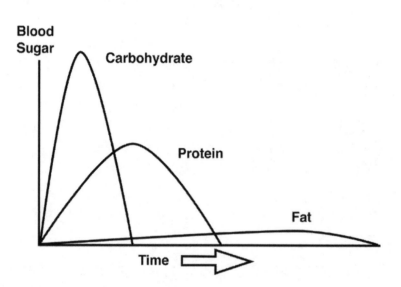

Remember that insulin and blood sugar levels work in parallel. When one is high, the other is high. With that said, from the above graph, we can see how carbohydrates, proteins, and fats affect blood sugar, thus insulin, levels over time. Of the three, the one that causes the greatest rise in blood sugar and insulin is carbs (and remember that carbs are synonymous with sugar). Next is protein at a moderate rate, and fats the lowest. If we disregard all that we have been taught in the past and we look at the science, we can see what we should eat. To lower the blood sugar levels and insulin production (which is what results in body fat), we should eat a lot of fat, a moderate amount of proteins, and just a few carbs. This may seem totally against what you have learned in the past, but if you remember what insulin does—it's the body's mechanism for causing sugar to be stored as body fat, among other things—then the science tells you something different. If what you did in the past hasn't worked, then you may have been trying, but just trying the wrong way.

When to Eat

8 Hour Eating Window
(16 hours fasting -- skipping breakfast)

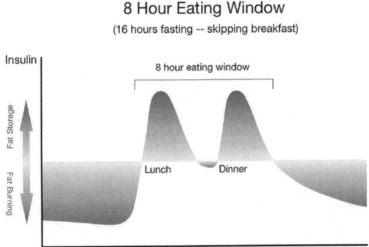

Look at the graph above and see how the timing of meals can affect insulin. Insulin is always being produced at a low level in a healthy individual. When we eat, the pancreas is stimulated and more insulin is then produced. After the insulin does its job to take the sugar and escort it to its destination (where it is either used by our brain, muscles, and body for energy; or taken to fat cells to be stored), the insulin returns at a low baseline.

If we look at the graph above, what do you think will happen then if we skip a meal? If we go more than 10 to 16 hours without food? What happens to the insulin? Insulin levels go down, and remember, when insulin is reduced, fat is not being stored. Do we just fall over if we skip a meal? No, the body has other ways of getting what it needs. This is where your body will begin to look for other sources of energy, and then your excess fat will be used for energy and weight loss will be augmented.

Most of us have been taught not to skip a meal. We were told that our metabolism would slow down and we would gain weight. But where is that evidence? I can't find it. But let's look at what we do know—if we don't eat, our insulin stays low. When we have low insulin, we have low fat storage.

So when do we eat? We eat when we are hungry. Once you start changing what you eat, things start to change on the inside. The hormones in your gut start to change—your hunger will go down and your satiety will go up. This is when you could start doing some mini-fasts. Fasts are simply going without any food or drink for a select amount of time—maybe 4 hours, maybe 8, 14, or 24 hours. Fasting will decrease your insulin levels, which is great because insulin is how fat storage happens—and that's what we want to avoid! I'm only mentioning mini-fasts now because they relate so well to insulin. In chapter 9 we'll explore intermittent fasting comprehensively.

Energy—Sugar-Burner or Fat-Burner?

Our bodies always need energy. Even when we are sleeping, energy is needed for breathing. When we are active, then more energy is needed. The hormonal system is always adjusting, trying to supply our body's needs. The body will get the energy it needs. If sugar is around, insulin is produced at a higher level and weight gain can occur. If sugar is not around, then your body adjusts and gets its energy from another source—your fat. This process of breaking down the fats for energy is called ketosis because the byproducts of fat are called ketone bodies. What we eat will affect where we get our energy. What we eat will affect our hormones.

At this point, you should be realizing that you are not what you eat. Eating fat will not make you fat. Skipping a meal will not wreck your metabolism. Your body is very complicated in some ways, but very simple in others. Having knowledge is key. Other hormones can affect you and your weight—such as your thyroid and adrenal hormones as well as your hunger hormone (ghrelin) and satiety hormone (leptin). For this book, however, just concentrating on insulin will help. Later, when we discuss the keto flu, come back and read this information again.

Why We Burn Sugar Instead of Fat

In our fat cells, we have energy stored as triglycerides. Our body can use this, but it has to break down the fat cells to get to the energy source. The key to activating this process is an enzyme called hormone sensitive lipase (HSL). An enzyme is a molecule needed for a process to occur. If the enzyme is not around or is inactive, the process will not happen. In our example, if HSL is around and active, it can be used to break down the fat cell for energy. However, guess which hormone makes this enzyme ineffective?

Insulin.

If our insulin is elevated, then HSL doesn't work quite right and the fat cell remains intact and can't be broken down for energy. High levels of insulin mean fat cells can't be used for energy. So, if your body needs energy, where does it go to first?

Sugar.

Sugar may give us energy, but the fat cells remain intact. Your body is using up the available sugar but can't break down the fat cell if more energy is needed because your insulin is preventing that reaction from happening. This leads to you wanting more sugar because you still need energy. This is also why you seem to be hungry even though you may be overweight, which presents another reason why having high levels of insulin is not good for you.

Now that you know how the body gets its energy in a typical diet, in the next chapter we dive into how the body gets its energy from a ketogenic diet—and why it's such an advantage when you aim to lose excess fat.

Billy H.'s Statistics

Billy is a 67-year-old male who started our plan in December 2017. His A1c, average blood sugar, was 13.4 (normal is less than 6.0), his triglycerides were 280 (ideally they should be less than 150), and his HDL, good cholesterol, was 22 (ideally it should be greater than 40). Then, four months in this plan, his A1c was 6.3, his triglycerides were 164, and his HDL was 31. Wow—talk about healthy improvements!

You don't have to be great to start, but you have to start to be great.

—Zig Ziglar

Chapter 5
An Intro to the Ketogenic Lifestyle

A ketogenic lifestyle is a dietary plan that minimizes the carbohydrate intake in a person's daily diet. In particular, a keto diet is a high-fat, low-carb, and moderate-protein diet. As you'll soon see, eating a ketogenic diet puts the body into ketosis—which is key for burning excess fat and getting the body into a very healthy state. In this chapter we'll explore what happens inside the body when you're eating a ketogenic diet as well as the many resulting health benefits.

Inside the Body:
From Sugar-Burning to Fat-Burning

The ketogenic dietary plan works on reducing the body's secretion of insulin, which is required for the absorption of food. Without insulin, the body is compelled to get its energy requirements by burning fat molecules, which would otherwise be stored in the body tissues as fat deposits (remember, chapter 4 covers this). By burning the intake of fats as well as the fat reserves in the body, weight loss is achieved.

The ketogenic lifestyle is scientifically proven to be successful and healthy. This is because proteins and fats—not carbohydrates—are the only macronutrients essential for body growth and development. An essential food is one that we have to take in by our diet because the body cannot produce them itself.

On the other hand, carbohydrates are a nonessential food, meaning that your body can produce them if needed, and they can be significantly reduced in the daily diet plan without causing a real impact on the overall health. Eating vast amounts of carbohydrates isn't necessary for the body to function, and when we do eat them, they cause insulin to increase (so fat doesn't get burned). For these two reasons we can avoid carbohydrates and get most of our energy from eating fats and proteins. Fats and proteins will supply our body with the energy it needs to function and at the same time will allow us to burn our fat reserves and keep our body weight at low and healthy levels. This is the reasoning behind the ketogenic diet's focus on fats and proteins.

Why is this diet called "ketogenic"? Let me explain. When a person has a low carbohydrate intake, their glucose (sugar from carbs) levels and secretion of insulin are also low. Once the body is relying on fats for energy (rather than carbohydrates), the burning of fats releases small fuel molecules known as ketones.

The process of producing ketones is known as ketosis. This diet is called "ketogenic" because by following the diet's recommendations on what and when to eat, you end up putting your body in ketosis. Ketosis is a good thing. It's the whole point of the diet. Ketosis simply means that your body derives energy from excess fat rather than from glucose (or carbohydrates).

When people talk about a low-carb diet, most immedi-ately think of the Atkins diet. While this is low carb, it contains many more grams of protein than what the ketogenic diet recommends. Let's recall chapter 4, where we learned that protein, while not as much as carbs, still stimulates insulin, which we are trying to control. This is why we don't want to eat lots and lots of protein on the ketogenic diet.

You'll see that the ketogenic diet recommends increas-ing your fat intake, but doesn't recommend increasing your fatty protein intake. Some of your fat will come from proteins, but not all. For example, you can't eat more hamburger with the goal of increasing your fats because the more hamburger you eat, the more you are also increasing your proteins. So to increase your fat intake, turn to the foods containing only the fat you need (without a protein overload): olive oil, butter, sour cream, or cream cheese. And don't worry—I'll help you identify fats, proteins, and fatty proteins in this book. You won't have to figure it out yourself!

The other term used in the diet world is "calories." If you haven't noticed, we haven't discussed counting calories in regard to the ketogenic diet. We are concerned with what type of foods you are eating, not the quantity. Obviously, if you take in 7,000 calories, no matter what you are eating, you will gain weight. At some point, if weight gain is stalled, you may have to look at the number of calories you are taking in, but, so far, this hasn't come up with any of the many people I've been guiding in the ketogenic plan.

Again, you will learn what and when to eat. Eating the prescribed foods will affect your hormones in a positive way getting you to the point where you will feel full and not go hungry.

Benefits of the Keto Diet

There are several benefits that can be achieved with a ketogenic lifestyle. Let's take a look at those to further convince you to commit to this lifestyle.

1 Weight Loss

To begin with, following a low-carb diet has been proven to cause significant weight loss, due to forcing the body to burn its fat reserves, rather than sugars and carbohydrates, to produce the required energy. Getting rid of the fat reserves simply means weight loss. In addition, burning fats instead of carbohydrates helps you to feel less hungry and, hence, is very useful in controlling the appetite.

One added point: before starting, I recommend that you measure your waist (I wish I had done this before I started!). Once you commit to the ketogenic lifestyle, not only will you see the numbers on the scale go down, you will see the notches in your belt change as well—this means you are losing fat rather than muscle!

2 More Energy

Moreover, by burning fats, the body produces higher energy in comparison to burning similar volumes of carbohydrates. As already explained, once the body is relying on fats for energy (rather than carbohydrates), the burning of fats releases small fuel molecules known as ketones. The process of producing ketones is known as ketosis. Ketosis helps in regulating the acidity of the body. As your body starts to change from a sugar burner to a fat burner—so as it readjusts itself and goes into ketosis—you will see an increased amount of energy. The fat seems to be a "cleaner fuel," a fuel that your body uses more efficiently.

3 Improved Brain Function

Prolonged adoption of a ketogenic lifestyle also helps in improving brain functionality as compared to extensive sugar consumption. This is because, when the body depends on sugar for fuel, certain reactive oxygen molecules are produced. Accumulation of these molecules due to an increased intake of sugar is known to cause a buildup of plaque around the brain cells, which impairs brain functions.

A ketogenic diet avoids this circumstance by using ketones for energy instead of burning glucose. In this way, there's a reduction in the production of those reactive (bad) oxygen molecules, which means there's a reduction in the buildup of that plaque around the brain.

4 Improved Cholesterol

In addition to the above mentioned benefits, a ketogenic diet is also found to be useful in regulating cholesterol levels in the body, which ultimately reduces the risk of heart diseases. Studies into the effect of high-fat low-carb dietary plans reveal that these diets can increase the levels of the beneficial HDL cholesterol. In addition, while it does not reduce the production of the harmful LDL cholesterol, a ketogenic diet changes the structure of the LDL cholesterol molecules such that their risks can be reduced. By regulating the levels of cholesterol in the body, a keto diet can potentially provide cardiovascular benefits and potentially reduce the risk of heart disease.

5 Lower Glucose and Triglycerides

As discussed before, a lower glucose/insulin level will lead to a lower fat level. Not only will this lead to weight loss, but your overall health will improve. Diabetics can expect a lower glucose level and even a possible lowering of medication. Remember that if you are a diabetic discuss the possibility of adjusting your medications with your medical provider before making any changes.

Disease Treatment and Keto

Obesity—following from our discussions so far, the key disease that is treated with a ketogenic diet is obesity. A high-fat and low-carb diet forces the body to burn excess body fat to generate its energy requirements. This, in turn, both reduces the fat reserve in the body and introduces a feeling of fullness that encourages you to eat less because you feel less hungry.

Diabetes—although medical consultation and supervision are required for diabetic patients before they follow a ketogenic diet, it is known to be particularly useful for patients with type 2 diabetes as it helps reduce the risk of many of its associated complications.

Type 2 diabetes is caused due to insulin resistance such that the body is unable to utilize the insulin it is secreting. In the ketogenic diet, by eating mostly fats and proteins, you end up lowering your insulin secretion. This then is significantly useful in limiting the severity of your insulin resistance. In fact, it can improve your insulin sensitivity, thereby reducing the chances of occurrence of type 2 diabetes.

Epilepsy—another disease that can be treated with a ketogenic diet is epilepsy, particularly in children. Several studies have been conducted since 1924 to today that monitor the effect of following a ketogenic diet on children who have epilepsy with frequent seizures.

In particular, studies conducted in 1924, 1998, and in our current decade, have all shown a significant improvement in epilepsy in children who pursued the ketogenic diet for 3 months, 6 months, and a full year. The results have mainly been an over 90% decrease in the frequency of seizures, which is a better effect compared to several other conventional therapies. Needless to say, before adopting this diet medical consultation and supervision remain essential to be able to monitor and analyze the results carefully.

Alzheimer's—as mentioned in the section about "Improved Brain Function," because the ketogenic diet stimulates the body to go into ketosis so that the body uses ketones as energy sources, this, in turn, helps to protect the neuron cells of the brain from plaque buildup. This means that it reduces chances of neuron cell impairments, which helps to improve the brain's cognitive performance. This was particularly evident in studies that investigated the effect of a ketogenic diet on Alzheimer's patients. These studies found ketone production improves the memory functions for Alzheimer's patients, so it might be able to reverse this disease.

Cancer—the ketogenic diet is also found to be one of the most suitable dietary plans for cancer patients. This is because, for one, it deprives cancerous cells of their main source of energy, which is sugar, thereby hin-dering their growth and slowing down their division rates. The second reason is that the low-carbohydrate intake in a keto diet reduces the production of a molecule named insulin-like growth factor (IGF-1), which is associated with the development of cancerous cells. Hence, although a ketogenic diet would not be the sole treatment for cancer, it complements the treatment process and helps in reducing the activity of cancerous cells.

Who Should Proceed with Caution?

The health benefits achieved by adopting this diet as a lifestyle reveal its general safety for the human body. Nevertheless, people with some health conditions still need to consult their doctors before pursuing a keto diet. Who needs to be cautious when following a keto diet? People with diabetes, people with high blood pressure, women who are pregnant or breastfeeding, and people who have had their gallbladders removed. I'll explain the groups individually below.

People diagnosed with diabetes should consult their physicians before beginning a ketogenic diet. In spite of the benefits of the ketogenic diet in controlling type 1 diabetes' complications and reversing the effect of type 2 diabetes, diabetics should seek proper medical consultation before adopting this dietary plan. Why? Because this diet directly influences blood glucose levels and, hence, the secretion of insulin. A consultation with a doctor will ensure that this dietary plan won't cause any side effects that may hinder the treatment process.

High blood pressure and pregnancy or breastfeeding are also conditions that need medical supervision if a keto diet is to be followed. This is because the body's requirement for nutrients differ during these conditions, and the proportional intake of macronutrients (meaning fat, protein, and carbohydrates) would need to be adjusted to address the body's demand for regulating blood pressure and for providing the necessary nutrients for baby growth during gestation and breast-feeding.

People with their gallbladders removed may find it difficult to adopt a ketogenic lifestyle. This is because the bile secreted by the gallbladder is a key player in the digestion of fats and elimination of excess cholesterol. When there is no gallbladder and this bile is not secreted, it becomes difficult for the body to break down its fat intake. Nevertheless, if it is essential for a person without a gallbladder to go on a ketogenic diet, certain guidelines need to be followed.

To begin with, the body needs to learn to digest fats without a gallbladder. This requires a training period in which the person avoids high-fat and low-fiber meals until the body has adapted to its new digestion routine. It is best to start with easily digestible foods and a sufficient intake of liquids, then have smaller meals at frequent intervals throughout the day. High-fiber foods are also highly recommended as they stimulate the intestines and ease the food digestion and absorption processes. Bile supplements may also be needed in case a high-fat meal has been consumed.

In addition to the above guidelines, the person needs to make sure they are well hydrated with sufficient intake of potassium, sodium, and magnesium, and to consume ginger or ginger tea to improve fat digestion. Once the person finds that their body is able to digest moderate amounts of fat, the fat intake can be increased slowly, with the bile supplements in place, until a complete keto diet can be adopted.

To briefly review this chapter, you learned in the typical diet, in which a person gets most of their calories from carbohydrates, the body sends out insulin to take the sugar (glucose) from those carbohydrates to fuel the body's cells. The insulin also stores any sugar (glucose) that isn't needed by cells as fat on a person. By following the ketogenic diet, and getting most of your calories from healthy fats, you change this mechanism in your body to the point where it's another process providing the body with its fuel: ketosis. This is what we want because it doesn't involve insulin; thus, there's no fat getting stored. Instead, fat is getting burned—so you lose weight and keep it off! You also learned how the ketogenic diet results in overall improved health as well as aiding in the treatment of potential diseases and unwanted health conditions.

Now that you've learned how keto works and its benefits, the next chapter supplies the necessary information on food and eating, so you can eat according to the ketogenic diet—and get started losing weight immediately.

Carl S.'s Statistics

Carl was diagnosed with diabetes and was taking medication to treat the disorder. His A1c(average blood sugar) was markedly elevated at 11.8 (normal 6.0 or lower). After beginning this new ketogenic lifestyle, his A1c dropped to below normal at 5.8. Carl is a testament to the incredible improvement in health a ketogenic diet gives you access to!

References

https://www.dietdoctor.com/low-carb/keto#intro

https://www.dietdoctor.com/low-carb/recipes/vegetarian

https://www.ruled.me/benefits-ketogenic-diet/

https://www.ruled.me/how-to-follow-keto-without-a-gallbladder/

The way you live your life today is preparing you for tomorrow. The question is—what are you preparing for?

—Anonymous

Chapter 6
Ketogenic Dos and Don'ts—
Your Prescription for Success

As laid out in the previous chapter, the ketogenic diet relies on putting your body into ketosis. When this happens, your body changes from sugar-burning to fat-burning, so that you end up burning off any excess pounds you may be carrying. In order to get your body into ketosis, most of the food you'll be eating are fats and proteins. As promised in the previous chapter, you aren't going to be expected to figure out this stuff by yourself.

This chapter lays out all the dos and don'ts on what you should (and should not) be eating on the ketogenic diet. We start with an overview and then get down to particular foods. Expect lots of helpful lists. Also, we'll cover any special considerations in the keto diet, for example exercise and vegetarianism.

Again, I encourage you to go to www. ourketogeniclife.
com, so you can educate yourself even more on the ketogenic lifestyle and immerse yourself in a

community of people who, like you, are eager to learn and striving to thrive in the lifestyle. The more people you have on your team that you can exchange support, ideas, and enthusiasm with, the happier and more successful you'll be.

A Keto Overview

The key advice when starting a keto diet is to adopt its guidelines as a lifestyle, rather than a diet that you would pursue for a certain period of time and then stop. However, pursuing a ketogenic lifestyle does not mean that you will be deprived of your food desires. Rather, it is just that you'll need to be quite strict to begin with in order to get the body to switch from burning sugars to burning fats—which is ketosis. And you personally need to get used to eating a certain class of foods (which we discuss in detail in this chapter).

Later, once the body has adapted to this new routine and you've started losing weight, you will be able to introduce the foods you love—at certain times and in calculated amounts. In this way you can allow yourself to enjoy those certain super tasty foods while not losing the weight loss you have achieved.

The first step to getting started on the ketogenic diet is to calculate (1) your calorie intake carefully and (2) how much of those calories should be taken from the key macronutrients: fats, proteins, and carbohydrates.

The point is not to be counting your calories. I told you already that's not what happens in this diet. The point of making these calculations is to ensure you are eating the correct ratio of fat, protein, and carbs to put your body into ketosis, which makes it burn fat.

Since a ketogenic diet is a low-carb and high-fat diet, the percentage of calories taken in the form of carbohydrates is very low—as low as 5% of your total calorie intake. The ratio of calories to be taken from each of the main nutrients (macronutrients) in order to put your body into ketosis and keep it there is reflected in the table below:

Nutrient	Percentage from Total Required Calories
Fats	75%
Proteins	20%
Carbohydrates	5%

The overall calorie requirements of a person's body can be estimated as 10 times the person's weight in pounds. For example, a person weighing 200 pounds typically requires 2,000 calories daily because 200 x 10 is 2,000. Using the above percentages, these 2,000 calories can be divided into:

- **Fat**: 75% of 2,000 = 1,500 calories from fat. Fats ave 9 calories per gram, so 1,500 divided by 9 = 166 grams of fat eaten per day.

- **Protein**: 20% of 2,000 = 400 calories from protein. Protein has 4 calories per gram, so 400 divided by 4 = 100 grams of protein eaten per day.

- **Carbs**: 5% of 2,000 = 100 calories from carbohydrates. Carbs have 4 calories per gram, so 100 divided by 4 = 25 grams of carbohydrates eaten per day.

Remember that the percentages are the most important numbers to look at. I have given you an estimate as to the number of calories to take in. But if you are hungry, eat more while staying within the given percentages.

An example keto meal plan for a day can be as follows:

- Eggs with bacon for breakfast

- A cup of bone broth with chicken salad for lunch

- Steak with sautéed veggies for dinner

Although this might be a good low-carb and high-fat example, the possibilities are endless. Keto dietitians worldwide recommend various meal combinations. You can find great ketogenic meal ideas and share your own fabulous ketogenic meal plans with others in the online keto community found at www.ourketogeniclife.com.

Now that you have this information about the ratio of calories to be taken from each of the main nutrient groups, let's learn more about those nutrient groups. In the rest of this chapter, we'll take a deep dive into fat, protein, and carbohydrates, so you are well educated to enjoy the keto lifestyle to the fullest.

Fat and Oils Dos and Don'ts

In order to accurately plan the keto diet, you need to know the food groups that need to be eaten as well as the ones to be avoided in order to take the body into ketosis and keep it there. Let's start by looking at fats and oils.

Fats and oils constitute the largest percentage of the calorie intake during a keto diet, reaching up to 75% of your total calorie intake per day. However, different types of fatty products exist, so correct choices need to be made. For instance, the ketogenic diet needs to include foods that are rich in saturated fats, mono-unsaturated fats, and naturally occurring poly-unsaturated fats. These fats are known to be chemically stable and are less inflammatory when compared to trans fats, which you must completely avoid.

Balancing between omega-3 and omega-6 intakes is also very useful To gain these, you should aim to include fatty fish and animal meat in your diet.

Remember, good fats are your friend. Adding these fats will help you reach ketosis and become "fat adapted" (this is explained in chapters 3 and 10). Look to use these when cooking or on and in your food:

- Olive oil

- Coconut oil

- MCT oil

- Avocado oil

- Avocados

- Butter—real butter, preferably grass-fed

Most foods do not contain 100% one specific type of fat. They are usually a mix between two or more types. Let's look more at the three kinds of healthy fats: saturated fats, monounsaturated fats, and naturally occurring polyunsaturated fats.

Saturated fats—examples of saturated fats include real butter, red meat, cream, eggs, and coconut oil (which is an MCT oil). Increasing your HDL or good cholesterol is associated with a diet that is higher in saturated fats. These fats are solid at room temperature and can be used for cooking at high temperatures.

Monounsaturated fats—examples include olive oil, avocados and avocado oil, macadamia nuts, and lard. These are associated with a reduction in abdominal fat, improvement in cholesterol, and reduction of inflammation. They are liquid at room temperature and are best for low-heat cooking.

Polyunsaturated fats—examples of these include walnuts, nut oils, and fatty fish like salmon. These fats include omega-3 and omega-6 fats, and are essential fats, meaning that we must consume them in our foods. Foods rich in omega-3 fats include salmon, avocados, walnuts, and olive oil. Foods rich in omega-6 fats include sunflower seeds, pistachios, and pumpkin seeds. A ratio of 1:1 of omega-3 and omega-6 fats are important to your diet—meaning we should eat equal amounts of both each day. However, the problem with the Western diet is that we eat too many omega-6 fats. For this reason, I recommend you concentrate on getting enough omega-3s, even taking a supplement if needed.

Trans fats—these are to be avoided at all times if possible. Examples of these are the hydrogenated and processed vegetable oils that are found in margarine, cookies, and fast foods. These fats increase inflammation and can elevate your insulin levels. Since you can control what you eat when you fix meals at home and you cannot control how food is prepared in restaurants, this is another reason to cook at home and use the oils that you know are good for you.

Protein Dos and Don'ts

Proteins are important to include in the ketogenic diet, but remember that it is not an all-you-can-eat-protein lifestyle. We want to have a moderate intake of protein. If we take in too much protein, then our body will use the excess to create glucose. This process is called gluconeogenesis, which means a creation (genesis) of new (neo) glucose (sugar/carbs). The ketogenic diet aims to get the body into ketosis to where it is fueling itself by burning fat; gluconeogenesis throws the body out of ketosis. In terms of protein intake, aim for taking in 20% of your total calories from protein sources. This will ensure you get the needed protein and also stay in ketosis.

While you can choose any type of protein, remember you want to choose fatty, non-processed meats if possible. A grilled chicken breast is acceptable, but you will have to add fats like olive oil or sour cream to increase the fat content without adding to the protein count.

Here's a list of good protein sources:

- *Meat*: beef, veal, goat, wild game

- *Pork*: loin, butt, chops, shoulder

- *Ham*: make sure the ham isn't too high in carbs. Remember to read labels.

- *Bacon*: make sure it has 0 grams of carbs. Remember to read labels.

- *Sausage*: it should only have 1 gram of carbs. Remember to read labels.

- *Poultry*: chicken, turkey, cornish hen, duck

- *Fish or seafood*: anchovies, calamari, catfish, cod, flounder, halibut, herring, mackerel, mahi-mahi, salmon, sardines, scrod, sole, snapper, trout, shellfish, clams, crab, lobster, scallops, shrimp, squid, mussels, oysters, tuna (canned tuna or salmon is fine. Just make sure there's no sugar added.)

- *Whole eggs*

- *Natural almond butter*: no added sugars are acceptable

Vegetables Dos and Don'ts

Not all vegetables are equal; there are starchy and non-starchy vegetables. You want to eat non-starchy vegetables, which have lower carbs. Avoid starchy vegetables completely.

Below you'll find two lists. The first lists non-starchy vegetables as well as their carbohydrate content. The second lists starchy vegetables as well as their carbohydrate content. If you scan both lists, you can see that a serving of vegetables can vary widely in its carb content. If you are limiting your carbs to 20 grams per day, picking a starchy carb can increase that count very easily.

I recommend totally avoiding starchy vegetables and instead eating different types of non-starchy vegetables. Explore ones that you haven't tried in the past.   As   far as choosing the best ones, look for dark and leafy vegetables like spinach or kale. If you are at the store and can't remember which are allowed, look for cruciferous ones or vegetables that grow above the ground like broccoli, cauliflower, and cucumbers.

It is easy to include different vegetables in salad. You will be able to include ones that you haven't tried before and that may give a different taste. Also a nice way to include vegetables is to saute them in some olive or coconut oil.

Non-Starchy Vegetables

Description	Amount	Net Carbs (g)
Watercress, raw	1 cup	0.2
Green onions (tops only), raw	1 tbsp	0.2
Beet Greens,	1 cup	0.3

raw		
Lettuce (red leaf), raw	1 cup	0.3
Ginger root, raw	1 tsp	0.4
Spinach, raw	1 cup	0.4
Arugula, raw	1 cup	0.4
Broccoli raab, cooked	1 cup	0.5
Lettuce (romaine), raw	1 cup	0.6
Mustard greens, raw	1 cup	0.8
Broccoli (Chinese), cooked	1 cup	1.2
Lettuce (iceberg) raw	1 cup	1.2
Turnip greens, raw	1 cup	1.3
Tomatillos, raw	1 medium	1.4

Celery, raw	1 cup	1.4
Radishes, raw	1 cup	2
Savoy cabbage, raw	1 cup	2.1
Spinach (frozen), cooked	1 cup	1
Cauliflower, cooked	1 cup	2.1
Asparagus, raw	1 cup	2.4
Spinach, cooked	1 cup	2.5
Sauerkraut, canned	1 cup	2.6
Garlic, raw	1 tbsp	2.6
Zucchini (summer squash), raw	1 cup	2.7
Portabella mushrooms, grilled	1 cup	2.7
Green bell peppers, sautéed	1 cup	2.8

Jalapeno peppers, canned	1 cup	3
Zucchini (summer squash), cooked	1 cup	3
Collards, cooked	1 cup	3.1
Cucumbers (with peel), raw	1 cup	3.2
Cauliflower, raw	1 cup	3.2
Brown mushrooms	1 cup	3.2
(Italian or cremini), raw	1 cup	
Kale, raw	1 cup	3.5
Mustard greens, cooked	1 cup	3.5
Swiss chard, cooked	1 cup	3.5
Shiitake mushrooms, stir-fried	1 cup	3.6
Broccoli, raw	1 cup	3.6

Beet greens, cooked	1 cup	3.7
Asparagus, cooked	1 cup	3.8
Green chile peppers, canned	1 cup	4
Tomatoes, raw	1 cup	4
Artichokes (globe or French), cooked	1 medium	4
Green snap beans, raw	1 cup	4.3
Green bell peppers, raw	1 cup	4.4
Brussels sprouts, raw	1 cup	4.6
Red cabbage, raw	1 cup	4.7
Kale, cooked	1 cup	4.7
Turnips, cooked	1 cup	4.8
White mushrooms, cooked	1 cup	4.9

Red bell peppers, sautéed	1 cup	5.1
Yellow onions, sautéed	1 cup	5.3
Green snap beans, cooked	1 cup	5.9
Red bell peppers, raw	1 cup	5.9
Broccoli, cooked	1 cup	6
Turnips, raw	1 cup	6.1
Eggplant, cooked	1 cup	6.1
Crushed tomatoes, canned	1/2 cup	6.5
Peas, boiled	1 cup	6.8
Brussels sprouts, cooked	1 cup	7.1
Spaghetti squash (winter squash), cooked	1 cup	7.8

| Leek, cooked | 1 cup | 8.3 |

Starchy Vegetables (Avoid These Vegetables)

Description	Amount	Net Carbs (g)
Carrots, raw	1 cup	8.7
Pumpkin	1 cup	9.3
Beets	1 cup	13.5
Peas	1 cup	14
Butternut squash	1 cup, cubed	15
Acorn squash	1 cup, cubed	20
Corn on the cob	1 ear	22
Boiled white potato	1 medium potato	25
Corn kernels	1 cup	30
Baked sweet potato	1 large potato	31

Mashed potato	1 cup	34
Plantains	1 cup, sliced	44
Mashed sweet potato	1 cup	50

Beans and Legumes Don'ts

Avoid beans and legumes, at least until your goals are reached. While beans and legumes are high in fiber and protein, they contain a lot of carbs. Eating these will easily derail your progress in that they will throw the body out of ketosis. Later on, it may be possible to include these sparingly in your diet.

Examples of beans and legumes include black beans, kidney beans, garbanzo beans, chickpeas, and pinto beans. Avoid these and all beans and legumes.

Dairy Products Dos and Don'ts

With dairy go full fat. Because the success of the ketogenic diet depends on your body going into ketosis, the only way for that to happen is for you to consume most of your calories from fat. This means you'll need to choose full-fat dairy products, NEVER low-fat or fat-free dairy.

Avoid milk entirely. Milk is not allowed as a serving can contain up to 12 grams of sugar. Even worse are evaporated and condensed milks, which can contain up to 25 grams and 166 grams of sugar respectively.

Adding whipping cream and sour cream can be an excellent way to increase your fat intake without increasing your protein intake. By the way, whipping cream and sour cream are also great to make food taste so much better.

Make an effort to eat the following:

- Full-fat heavy whipping cream

- Hard and soft cheeses

- Full-fat cream cheese

- Full-fat cottage cheese (in moderation. A quarter-cup has around 2 grams of carbs)

- Full-fat Greek yogurt (beware of added sugars, and eat in moderation)

- Full-fat sour cream (make sure it doesn't contain more than 1 gram of carbs per serving)

Nuts and Seeds Dos and Don'ts

Nuts and seeds, especially roasted ones, represent a great source of fats. However, consume them with care as they may also be high in carbohydrates, which defies the purpose of the keto diet. They also contain protein, which should be acknowledged in calculating your daily total protein intake, to avoid an excessive intake.

The most preferred nuts in a keto diet are fatty low-carbohydrate nuts such as macadamia nuts, Brazil nuts, and pecans. Moderate carbohydrate nuts such as walnuts and almonds can be moderately included to supplement the dietary plan. Pistachios and cashews should be completely avoided as they have much higher carbohydrate contents and would disturb the keto diet plan.

Below you'll find a list of nuts and seeds, and their corresponding fat, protein, and calories.

Nutritional Values of Nuts and Seeds per 1 Ounce

	Approx # of Nuts	Total Fat	Total Protein	Total Calories
Almonds	23	14	6	160
Brazil Nuts	6	19	4	190
Hazelnuts (filberts)	21	17	4	180
Macadamia Nuts	11	22	2	200

Pecans	19 halves	20	3	200
Pine Nuts	165	20	4	190
Pistachios	49	18	4	160
Walnuts	14 halves	18	4	190
Chia Seeds		9	4	139
Flax Seeds		12	5	151
Pumpkin Seeds		13	7	153
Sesame Seeds		14	5	162
Sunflower Seeds		14	6	162

Water and Beverages

Drinking water is essential for all people across all age groups, but the requirements when on a keto diet tend to increase slightly. This is because a high-fat and low-carb diet inherently has a diuretic effect, which may lead to dehydration. Hence, increasing the intake of water from the recommended 8 glasses per day to around a gallon per day helps to avoid potential dehydration. Drinking water throughout the day will help you avoid feeling tired and also decrease food cravings. Water will aid in digestion as well.

While moderate drinking of tea and coffee is recommended, soda and alcohol consumption should be significantly reduced or even eliminated from your diet, mainly due to their high sugar content.

Don't drink your calories. I've had several patients start the keto diet at this point, simply by stopping their consumption of all soft drinks. The weight will drop off at the beginning, and you will see results in a week or two. Try to avoid all alcohol as well. All alcohol is a toxin to your body and can affect your liver. When you drink alcohol, the production of ketones will be lower.

Coffee is fine as long as you do not add sugar to it. Try to put MCT oil, butter, or heavy cream in your coffee. It may take some time, but eventually if you decide to add intermittent fasting (discussed in detail in a later chapter) and not eating breakfast to your ketogenic lifestyle, then drinking black coffee is a great way to continue your fast.

If you have to have a sweet cup of tea, use stevia as a sugar substitute. If you have to have a fizzy drink, there's company called La Croix that makes no-calorie, flavored seltzer waters.

Fruits

When you begin the ketogenic diet, hold off from eating any fruit. While fruits do provide nutrients, you want to hold off any excess sugar intake until your goals are reached.

The sugar in fruits is called fructose, which is metabolized in a different way than glucose (sugar from carbs) is metabolized. Fructose is metabolized through the liver. If you have an excess of glucose (sugar from carbs), any fructose (from fruit you've eaten) is stored as fat in your liver. The body can use this fructose stored as fat in your liver later for energy if needed. If we are storing more fructose than we are using, it can lead to a condition called fatty liver disease. Don't worry, in the ketogenic lifestyle, you will get to the point where you can reintroduce fruit, but wait until you reach your goals.

Carbohydrate Content of Allowed Fruits

Fruit	Amount	Total Carbs (g)	Fiber (g)	Net Carbs (g)
Lemon juice	2 tbsp	2	0	2

Lime juice	2 tbsp	2	0	2
Rhubarb	1 cup	2	2	4
Blackberries	1 cup	14	5	6
Raspberries	1 cup	15	5	7
Clementines	1 fruit	9	0	8
Cranberries	1 cup	19	2	8
Asian pear	1 sm. fruit	13	4	9
Strawberries	1 cup	12	3	9

Once our goals are reached, start with the above fruits—they are lower in carbs and will less likely prevent weight gain.

Artificial Sweeteners

Remember, our goal is to get off carbs (sugar) and eat more natural, non-processed foods. However, I know that we all will face the question of which sweetener to use when you want some sweetness in a recipe or drink. This is where a little education will be effective and help steer you in the right direction.

One way to measure which sweetener to choose is by using the glycemic index (GI). The GI measures how a food raises the blood sugar. For the ketogenic diet, the lower the GI, the better. To take this one step further, let's also consider how food affects your insulin level. The lower the insulin response, the better. The last factor that I look at is where the sweetener originated. The more we see a product coming from a natural source, as opposed to a laboratory-made chemical, the better.

Stevia—this is a natural extract from the herb Stevia rebaudiana. Stevia is 200 times sweeter than regular sugar, contains no carbs, and has zero calories. Stevia is the best sweetener to use and comes in a powder or liquid form.

Erythritol—this is a naturally occurring sweetener that does not affect your blood sugar. It can be used in many baked goods and is low in calories.

Inulin—this is another natural based sweetener that should not be confused with insulin. This sweetener can also be used in many baking recipes but has more calories than erythritol.

Sweetener	GI	Type	Net Carbs (per 100g)	Calories (per 100g)
Stevia	0	Natural	5	20

Erythritol	0	Sugar Alcohol	5	20
Inulin	0	Natural	1	150
Monk fruit	0	Natural	0–25	0–100
Xylitol	13	Sugar Alcohol	60	240
Maltitol	36	Sugar Alcohol	67	270
Sucralose	0–80	Artificial	0	0
Aspartame	0	Artificial	85	352
Saccharin	Variable	Artificial	94	364
Table sugar	63	Processed	100	387

Eating Out

Cooking at home is much preferred for maintaining the ketogenic lifestyle. When you cook at home, you can control not only what you eat but also how you prepare your food. Even still, we all know at some point we will be eating out, so we will need to make some educated decisions.

The one thing I would encourage you to do is to go online and check out the nutritional values of the food the restaurant is offering. Don't accept the excuse that you didn't know what you were eating and just plunged and ordered anything on the menu. Take control of your decisions and don't let your circumstances dictate your choices.

Following the ketogenic lifestyle may be quite challenging if you are used to having meals with friends outside the home or you go to many parties, meetings, or other events where you are offered a food menu rich in carbohydrates and a dessert menu full of sweets. Nevertheless, a good understanding of the requirements of a ketogenic lifestyle will help you decide on what to eat on these occasions and how far you can enjoy the available options without ruining what you have achieved so far with your keto diet.

The key recommendation when eating out is to minimize eating carbohydrate-loaded food! As plain as it may sound, this actually means that you can enjoy a juicy beef burger with vegetables but without eating the bun and skipping the fries platter altogether. Lettuce wraps are, in fact, quite common, and they are offered by several restaurants either as part of the menu or with a special request. Although a bun-less burger may sound discouraging, keep in mind that you are trying to build a balance between the healthy ketogenic lifestyle with its multiple benefits to your body and your desire to enjoy your time with friends at a fast food restaurant while being the odd one out.

Many restaurants now offer interesting salad mixes with different dressings to encourage people to stay healthy while having a delicious plate. After all, the salad does not have to be all green! A good mix of chicken or beef strips, lettuce, cheese, and sour cream, with some low-carb salad dressing can be a good option if you are afraid to ruin your dietary plan.

Breakfast meals outside the home that follow the ketogenic guidelines are the easiest and most common to find, as they simply need to include eggs, meat, bacon or turkey, and cheese—the common components of a breakfast plate anyway. This means that you are only skipping the bread and jam. Undoubtedly, you would also need to avoid any fried items such as French fries, fried chicken strips, or any fried vegetables.

While it might be quite challenging, to begin with, these recommendations will help you satisfy your body's craving for fast food and make it easier to follow your keto diet plan without feeling left out of important socializing occasions.

Fast Food—most fast food places offer a hamburger or chicken sandwich with fries. Some places like Hardee's and In-N-Out Burger offer a low-carb option by replacing a bun with a lettuce wrap. If you are in a restaurant that doesn't, then all you need to do is order the grilled chicken or any hamburger, and remove the bun. Then switch out your fries with a salad, decline any croutons, add your full-fat dressing, and you've got yourself a low-carb, high-fat dinner.

Salads—this is a great option, and you usually can order one at most any restaurant. Watch out for the hidden carbs in croutons, corn, and dried fruits. Don't be afraid to go full fat with the dressing, but look for an olive oil dressing if possible. Add some grilled chicken or even ask for a hamburger patty on the side.

Mexican—options here include ordering a plate of protein—shrimp, chicken, steak—and having a cheese sauce on the side. Tell the waiter to not bring the chips to the table and to hold the tortillas that usually come with meals. Adding a side of guacamole is a great way to add fat to your meal as well.

Asian—most everything here will include some sort of sauce or breading. Having a dry protein with a salad is probably the best option. If a Hibachi-type grill is available, a good option is to choose some proteins with vegetables.

Steaks—always go for a fatter type steak like a rib-eye or T-bone. Add a salad with vegetables. This is usually the easiest choice to make when deciding what type of restaurant to go to.

Pasta—ask to take off the pasta and serve your meal on a bed of vegetables. Watch out for hidden sugars in the sauces and tell them to hold the bread.

On Spices

Although it might be quite unexpected, spices do have carbohydrates in them. Hence, their intake must be regulated in order to follow a keto diet. If only a few spices are being used in the recipe, you do not have to worry about it. The problem will only arise if multiple spices are used, as their carbohydrate content would add up.

Know Your Weaknesses

We all have something that we have difficulty avoiding. That we are very susceptible to. For me, it's chocolate chip cookies. A platter full of cakes and pastries could be placed in front of me, and I wouldn't be tempted to eat them. But if you put cookies on that platter, I will eat each and every one . . . until they are *all* gone.

Your Achilles heel will be different—a type of food, the check-out lane at the grocery store, that bag of chips in your cabinet. You know what you're susceptible to.

In starting the ketogenic lifestyle, you will need to avoid and remove the temptation. Know though that it doesn't mean you'll never get to eat it for the rest of your life, just for now.

Be prepared for strong sugar cravings. The reason is that sugar tends to be quite addictive as it releases dopamine, the "happiness hormone," into the body, which then makes the body dependent on this secretion. In order to control sugar cravings, it is essential to have a strong will to eliminate sweeteners completely for the first 30 days until the body overcomes its desire for dopamine. This means that you need to clean out your house, car, and workspace, removing any sugary foods, to help keep your cravings controlled.

The body sometimes craves certain food because of a lack of certain nutrients. If these nutrients can be supplied using a healthy ketogenic food item, the craving can be significantly controlled. Use the following information to help you if you have any of these cravings:

- If you find you crave chocolate, the body may be in need of magnesium, which can be alternatively provided by eating nuts and/or seeds.

- Cravings for sugary food can be satisfied by eating cheese, chicken, or even broccoli because they contain chromium, carbon, phosphorus, and sulphur—the same nutrients found in sugary foods.

- Cravings for bread, pasta, and carbohydrates, in general, can be satisfied using high protein meat as it is a good source of nitrogen, a nutrient also found in bread and pasta.

- Salty foods, on the other hand, can be replaced with fish, nuts, and seeds in order to provide the body's requirements for chloride and silicon, nutrients also found in salty foods.

Special Considerations

The rest of this chapter addresses special considerations in regard to the ketogenic lifestyle. You will learn about the keto flu, vegetarianism and keto, and women on the keto diet. In chapter 7 we'll look at supplements and keto, and in chapter 8 we'll focus on exercise and keto. Remember, the more educated you are about the intricacies of the ketogenic lifestyle, the more you set yourself up for success—that's why I'm sharing these special considerations with you.

Keto Flu

When you start the ketogenic lifestyle, at the beginning, you may experience what we refer to as the keto flu. Simply put, you may feel sluggish, tired, and have no energy. There is a very good reason that this is happening. It is because your body is changing from burning sugar to burning fat for energy. Your body is adjusting internally. It is going into ketosis. For some people, this internal adjustment results in the keto flu.

The keto flu's effect is short term, lasting one to two weeks. Most people don't experience it, but I want to warn you in case you do.

How do you combat the keto flu? Here's the keto flu remedy: drink plenty of water and take in salt as well as some magnesium and potassium. You might need to take a magnesium supplement. If you follow the food guidelines given in this chapter, the magnesium and potassium will be in the foods you eat, such as avocados, dark green leafy vegetables, nuts, seeds, fatty fish, and meats. Just continue to drink water and add salt to your foods. That will usually take care of the symptoms. In the next chapter about supplements and keto, we'll talk more about how certain supplements can alleviate keto flu symptoms.

One week after one of my patients began the ketogenic lifestyle—let's call her Katia—Katia returned to my clinic to tell me she couldn't keep doing it. She explained that she felt very tired. I reminded her that this was the keto flu and that it would pass. Also, I encouraged her to apply the flu remedies. She agreed to continue the diet and take the remedies. A week later, Katia notified me to say she was feeling well and full of energy.

Vegetarianism and Keto

The vegetarian ketogenic diet, as suggested by the name, is a dietary plan that combines both the vegetarian and the ketogenic lifestyles, by following a plan that is free of meat, fish, and poultry while restricting the intake of carbohydrates. This diet, as it is not strictly vegan, allows the intake of eggs and dairy products, which will provide the necessary intake of proteins and fats required for a keto diet.

In order to implement vegetarian ketogenic diet, you need to significantly limit your intake of carbohydrates and build the plan on low-carb vegetables. These include leafy greens such as spinach; above-ground vegetables such as broccoli and cauliflower; and avocados and berries.

More importantly, however, you must have a sufficient intake of high-fat eggs and dairy products to provide the necessary fat intake, along with other healthy fats from olive oil and coconut oil.

Vegetarian-friendly protein sources are also very important in a vegetarian ketogenic diet, in order to supply the body's requirements for protein. These include tofu and tempeh, which are soy-based; and seitan, which is a vegetarian meat-substitute made of wheat gluten. Nuts and seeds can also provide a good source of protein, but you need to be careful about the carbohydrate content of these as some are high in carbs, such as pumpkin seeds, flax seeds, and pistachios.

Women and Keto

While most studies on ketogenic diets have involved men (or mice!) as experiment samples, most scientists have confidently stated that the ketogenic lifestyle would work equally well for females. Later studies on females who follow the ketogenic diet have enforced this conclusion, particularly with the observed weight loss, efficient blood sugar control, and enhanced sleep quality, as well as other benefits for women who are in their menopause stage.

However, certain side effects have been experienced by women who follow a ketogenic diet. These include bad breath, menstruation issues, constipation, and thyroid issues. These side effects can be considered exaggerated versions of the keto flu, which may be experienced at early stages of the ketogenic diet but tends to stop or significantly reduce after a few weeks. Quality sleep, plenty of water, and normal exercising can help reduce these side effects.

It is important for pregnant or breastfeeding women, as well as those with irregular menstrual cycles, to consult their doctors before following a ketogenic lifestyle.

Keto Dos-and-Don'ts Summary

To make it easier for you to follow a ketogenic diet, the first step is to learn to avoid or significantly reduce the intake of the following:

- *Sugar*—in the form of anything processed and sweet, such as soda, sports drinks, candy, and chocolate, particularly milk chocolate and white chocolate. Dark chocolate with 70% to 85% cocoa can occasionally be consumed without causing a severe impact.

- *Grains*—such as any wheat products, pasta, cereals, cakes, and pastries. This also includes whole wheat grains although they are perceived to be healthier.

- *Starch and starchy vegetables*—such as potatoes and yams. Oats and muesli should also be avoided.

- *Trans fats*—in margarine and other spreadable butter replacements

- *Fruits*—particularly large fruits that are high in sugars, such as apples, oranges, and bananas

- *Low-fat foods*—as they are likely to be very high in carbohydrates to substitute for the low-fat content

Remember too the fat-protein-carbs percentages. Most of your calories each day should come from fat: 75% to be exact. Next is protein at 25%. Finally, 5% of your calories can come from carbohydrates. When you eat in this ratio, you put your body in ketosis so that it burns excess fat (rather than sugar, which is what's burned in a carbohydrate-heavy diet). Ketosis is what we're looking for in the ketogenic lifestyle!

The First Steps

Remember I told you to take baby steps? You can find a list of starting steps at www.ourketogeniclife.com, and I'm offering them here as well:

1. Know your why and your specific goals. Write it all down.

2. Identify your weaknesses.

3. Bring the food list (located in chapter 13) with you to the grocery store.

4. Download an app to help you track your fat, protein, and carb intake to ensure you are eating the correct ratio to achieve and maintain ketosis. I use a free app called MyFitnessPal.

5. Limit your carbs to 20 grams or less per day (if you can't, try to do less than 50 grams).

6. Eat fat, trying to get 75% of your total daily calories from it.

   Note: when we try to increase our fat intake, the one way we can't do it is by increasing our fatty proteins. For example, we can't eat more hamburger with the goal being to increase our fat intake because the more hamburger we eat to increase our fat intake, the more we increase our protein intake as well. So, to increase our fat intake we turn to the foods containing only the fat we need: olive oil, butter, sour cream, or cream cheese.

7. Fill in the rest of the foods you need by eating proteins. Warning—don't take in an excess amount, as an excess will stimulate your insulin at too high levels.

8. As time goes on, listen to your body.

9. Start intermittent fasting, which we'll examine in chapter 9.

To help you start and to give you daily guidance, go to www.ourketogeniclife.com. The ketogenic community on the site, including me and my team, will guide you through the process. We can start you on a 21-day challenge, and I guarantee you will see results.

Remember, that a lifestyle of getting into ketosis is the key to weight loss, and low carbs are the key to getting into ketosis.

Leon M.'s Message

"I'll be honest; I've tried so many methods to lose weight and failed, but [the ketogenic] lifestyle is

absolutely the easiest thing I've ever done. The list of foods [see chapter 13] helps tremendously."— November 2017

References

https://www.perfectketo.com/keto-macro-calculator/

https://www.shape.com/fitness/tips/things-you-need-know-about-exercising-keto-diet

https://dietingwell.com/keto-diet-fast-food/

https://bioketo.com/mct-oil-ketosis-guide/

https://shop.bioketo.com/products/core-bhb-salts

https://draxe.com/hub/keto-diet/keto-diet-women/

*So . . . whether you eat or drink, or whatever you do,
do All for the Glory of God.*

—1 Corinthians 10:31

Chapter 7
Supplements and Keto

Changing to a ketogenic lifestyle involves teaching the body to derive its energy mostly from fats. The body has to make adjustments as it goes into ketosis where it becomes fat-burning rather than sugar-burning. As you learned already, for some people this one-to two-week adjustment period results in a keto flu.

To ease this transition many people like to take some initial preparation steps to help them and their bodies get ready for the new ketogenic lifestyle and diet. These steps entail doing cleanses and taking supplements. That's what we'll look at in this chapter.

Colon Cleanse

For the ketogenic diet to be maximally effective and for your body to adapt quickly to ketosis, many people choose to do a colon cleanse. Cleansing the colon, which is the gastrointestinal tract, allows for maximum absorption of the new fat-concentrated diet, you'll be eating in the ketogenic diet. Over years of eating a carbohydrate-heavy diet it is possible that waste and toxins have built up in your colon or that harmful microorganisms have collected there. This can disrupt the digestive system's microbiome and also make the digestive system less effective in properly absorbing the nutrients found in the foods you eat.

There are numerous benefits associated with a colon cleanse. The most important is the fact that a cleanse can help to improve the general function of the digestive system. Additionally, a cleanse can help to reduce your risk of becoming constipated. It's also been linked to higher levels of energy. When a ketogenic diet is followed to assist with weight loss, a colon cleanse becomes even more important. This is because cleansing the digestive tract can help to "kickstart" the body's metabolism.

The best way to cleanse the colon is to do so with the help of a supplement. There are a lot of different supplements that can be used to help cleanse the gastrointestinal tract and improve digestive function. Let's take a look at some of these supplements.

Cape aloe—cape aloe is a fairly popular supplement when it comes to colon cleanses. This is a type of aloe vera plant that is known to possess many healing properties that can aid in improving skin health, as well as the well-being of the internal body.

Senna leaves—senna leaves are one of the most popular natural laxatives on the market today. They are known to be both safe and effective for cleansing the digestive system, as well as aiding in relieving certain gastro-intestinal symptoms, such as constipation. Senna leaves can be bought loose and brewed up into a tea, or can be purchased in the form of a dietary supplement.

Cascara sagrada—this is another natural laxative that is effective in relieving constipation. It is often also used as a way to naturally clean out the digestive system. Supplements containing cascara sagrada should only be used for a short while—no longer than a single week—as side effects may occur when it is taken over longer periods of time. Such side effects may include muscle weakness and heart problems. Additionally, electrolyte levels may decline, such as levels of sodium, magnesium, chloride, and potassium.

Fennel seed—fennel seed extracts have many health benefits to offer the human body. The seeds are often used to make a tea that helps to ease gastrointestinal symptoms such as bloating. The tea is also a good way to relieve constipation. Thus, fennel seed supplements are sometimes used to cleanse the colon and improve overall digestion. The seed is also good for treating stomach cramps and flatulence. Fennel seed supplements may also be useful in reducing the presence of pathogenic bacterium species in the gastrointestinal tract.

African bird pepper—this spice is more commonly known as cayenne pepper. Supplements that contain this ingredient can help to reduce the symptoms associated with an upset stomach. It is also a good option for improving the function of the digestive system. The substance has been proven to help reduce intestinal gas, as well as to help eliminate toxins from the digestive tract.

These are not the only options to help detox your body and cleanse your digestive system. In addition to taking supplements, it is also a good idea to increase your intake of fiber as this would further help to clean out the colon.

Liver Cleanse

Some people detoxify their livers before they start the ketogenic diet. The liver is the organ in the human body that plays one of the most important roles in the ketogenic diet. Fats accumulates in the liver and is then converted into ketones by the liver. Thus, individuals who wish to follow this diet want to ensure their liver can quickly and effectively start to produce these ketones that will give them with energy.

A few natural compounds and supplements have been proven effective in helping to remove toxins from the liver and improve its overall function. Remember that when it comes to a liver cleanse, it is important to consider the particular supplements that you use and to follow the correct dosage. This will help to avoid possible harmful side effects from developing. Let's take a look at some of these supplements:

Dandelion—A particularly popular natural extract that is often used as an ingredient in a liver cleanse is dandelion, and it's often prepared as a tea. Dandelion may also be useful in improving digestive health and cleansing the colon. Furthermore, this natural extract may also help to ease an upset stomach, improve appetite, and treat joint pain. Some people have noted reduced muscle aches when drinking dandelion tea. Dandelion is also powerful against viral infections.

Glutathione—this is also another excellent option for cleansing the liver and removing toxins that might have built up in this vital organ. Glutathione is sometimes used in the treatment of liver disease due to the positive effects it has on this organ.

Ginger root—ginger root is popular for its antibacterial properties, and it has also been proven to be effective in cleansing the liver. Additionally, ginger root helps to detoxify the lymphatic system of the human body and is beneficial for the digestive system.

Milk thistle—milk thistle is probably one of the most popular natural ingredients associated with a liver cleanse. In addition to being useful in detoxifying the liver, milk thistle is often used in the treatment of jaundice, cirrhosis, and hepatitis. Some people also use it to treat gallbladder problems.

In addition to these particular supplements and natural extracts, there are other ways to help with the detoxification of the liver. Certain vitamins that have antioxidant properties, such as vitamin E and vitamin C, are known to help protect the liver against further damage. Selenium and zinc, two important minerals, also aid in improving liver function and protecting it against damage.

Supplements and Keto Flu

One negative that can happen to people starting the keto diet is the keto flu. We've mentioned it already, but let's look at it again briefly and then discuss the supplements that can remedy it.

On the ketogenic diet, you will reduce your carbohydrate consumption to 5% of your overall daily caloric intake and increase your fat consumption to cover 75% of your daily caloric intake. There are many changes that occur in the body during this process. The amount of insulin that is produced and secreted by the pancreas, for example, becomes lower. This is a good thing—as we've already discussed. The reduction in the secretion of insulin is the main reason why people start to follow this diet. It is the primary factor that leads to the diet's numerous benefits.

As insulin levels decline, fat is converted into compounds called "ketones" by the liver and the body relies on these ketones for its energy needs. At the stage where the body transitioned from using glucose for energy to fats, then a person is considered to be in "ketosis." While the body is going through this transition, keto flu often develops. The symptoms (to repeat them though we covered them in the previous chapter) can include fatigue, irritability, muscle cramps, dizziness, sugar cravings, brain fog, nausea, low levels of motivation, and headache. In the majority of cases, a person would only experience these symptoms for a couple of days. After they push through these symptoms, they will usually start to experience the benefits that a ketogenic diet can offer.

Know that the keto flu symptoms can interfere with your day-to-day activities. When you start to experience these symptoms, you may be less productive at work and find it difficult to get through the day. This is the common reason why people often add supplements to their lives when they start a ketogenic diet.

We start the supplement and keto discussion by looking at electrolytes that are always important to your body and that become even more important when the body transitions into ketosis. While it's possible to find these electrolytes in foods, many of these foods are carbo-hydrates, which you'll be eating only the smallest amount of. Because of this, consider opting for supple-ments to get your needed daily intake of the following electrolytes. Remember, my site   www.loveyournewyou. com offers keto-focused supplements for sale. Every

supplement I mention in this chapter is available at www.loveyournewyou.com. As a thank-you to my book readers, I'm offering a discount on your first order of supplements. Simply input the discount code BOOK
at www.loveyournewyou.com/book to receive the discount.

Sodium—the majority of individuals who want to get rid of keto flu symptoms as their body transitions toward a ketosis state first experiment with increasing their salt and water intake. The ketogenic diet can cause the body to become deprived of fluids quickly (i.e., diuretic). This also means sodium levels, as well as electrolyte levels, can quickly become low, thus resulting in muscle cramps. This is why muscle cramps are common among individuals who are just getting started with a ketogenic diet.

Simply drinking more water is a good way to increase fluids, but it is usually advised to increase salt intake too. This can often be accomplished by simply drinking water and eating foods that are higher in sodium. When the foods a person eats are low in sodium, they can simply add a pinch of salt to the food.

Electrolytes—Apart from salt and fluids, however, many people find that adding electrolyte supplements greatly helps them reduce the severity of keto flu symptoms. Electrolyte are also known as minerals. Electrolytes are essential for proper muscle and nerve function. In addition to the purpose that these minerals serve in allowing optimal muscle function and nerve impulses to be transmitted, electrolytes are also important for maintaining a balanced level of fluids in the body.

The following supplements are also important on a ketogenic diet to help avoid the symptoms that are often experienced during the first few days (keto flu):

Magnesium—magnesium is a very important mineral that is involved in the immune system, muscle function, nerve function, and in the maintenance of a healthy heart rate and rhythm. Together with another mineral, known as calcium, magnesium also helps to ensure bones are healthy. Over 300 functions in the body also depend on a healthy magnesium supply. Magnesium is also known to help regulate normal sleep cycles. In men, it contributes to the production of testosterone. Many foods contain high levels of magnesium, including leafy green vegetables, pumpkin seeds, avocados, and almonds. Men should try to obtain around 420 mg magnesium per day, and women should aim for around 320 mg of magnesium daily. It is vital to avoid taking too much magnesium, even when on a ketogenic diet, as this may lead to lethargy, an irregular heartbeat, urine retention, diarrhea, nausea, vomiting, muscle weakness, low blood pressure, and other symptoms.

Potassium—potassium is another electrolyte that the body needs to ensure optimal regulation of fluids, as well as to regulate blood pressure levels. Potassium is also vital for maintaining a normal, "healthy" heart rate. Furthermore, this particular electrolyte is important for the digestive system as it is involved in the breakdown of carbohydrates. It is important to note that potassium assists in the production of proteins. The mineral is present in mushrooms, salmon, leafy green vegetables, avocados, and in certain nuts. The recommended daily intake of potassium is between 3,500 mg and 4,700 mg, depending on factors such as body weight and gender. It is important to keep to these guidelines. Overdosing on potassium can also cause some side effects, such as tiredness, heart palpitations, an irregular heartbeat, chest pain, nausea, and breathing problems.

Calcium—a lot of people who are new to the ketogenic diet tend to forget about just how important calcium is. Most people tend to associate calcium with bone health. While this is 100% correct as calcium is one of the most important nutrients for the maintenance of healthy bones, many fail to realize that this mineral has many other functions to play in the body. For example, calcium is vital for the maintenance of blood clotting. Calcium also contributes to normal muscle contractions. Calcium is readily available in dairy products, such as milk, broccoli, and fish. Other sources of calcium also exist. The daily recommended calcium intake varies between 1,000 mg and 2,500 mg. The specific require-ments for each individual depend on their gender and age. Taking too much calcium can cause side effects, such as bone pain, abdominal pain, constipation, depression, headaches, diarrhea, and confusion.

There are two particular reasons why people might want to consider obtaining an adequate supply of these particular electrolytes through supplements instead of only through food sources. Firstly, many of the foods that have high levels of calcium, potassium, and magnesium are also known to be high in carbohydrates (yes, even vegetables can contain an alarming amount of carbs as you know from our discussion on starchy vegetables!). When on a ketogenic diet, carbohydrate intake needs to be restricted; thus, it may not be possible to gain an adequate supply of these minerals, along with all other nutrients needed, only from whole food sources.

Tip: people who find it difficult to balance their intake of electrolytes when they are entering a state of ketosis can opt for bone broth. Bone broth is high in essential nutrients, particularly in electrolytes. Eating it helps to maintain normal levels of magnesium, potassium, and even sodium when on a ketogenic diet. Those individuals who usually buy low-sodium options of bone broth may also consider adding a little salt to the broth before consumption to help increase their intake of sodium. Sodium is also important for the maintenance of fluid, especially during the early stages of the ketogenic diet.

Vitamin D—Another factor that should be taken into consideration is that certain minerals require additional nutrients for optimal absorption. Calcium is the primary mineral to look at here. It requires vitamin D to be absorbed properly. The majority of calcium supple-ments on the market today already include an appropriate supply of vitamin D to ensure the calcium can be absorbed without any problems.

Vitamin D itself also plays a vital role in the ketogenic diet and the human body in general. This fat-soluble vitamin is not present in a lot of different foods, making it even harder to obtain an adequate supply when switching to a low-carb, high-fat diet. This is yet another reason why people opt for supplements.

When it comes to supplying the body with vitamin D, it is important for people to take note of the fact that most calcium supplements would only provide an adequate supply of vitamin D to ensure proper absorption of the calcium. This may not be enough to support all the functions that vitamin D contributes to in the human body. Thus, additional supplementation of this particular vitamin should be considered.

Vitamin D is also involved in the growth of cells, as well as in the regulation of inflammatory responses within the body. The vitamin is involved in the immune system. Furthermore, there is a significant number of cells in the body that contain receptors that respond to the presence of vitamin D.

The recommended daily vitamin D intake varies widely depending on the age of a person. Children and teens are advised to obtain around 400 IU of vitamin D per day. Adults, however, require approximately 2,000 IU of vitamin D every day. People who do not gain an adequate amount of sun exposure should consume more vitamin D in supplement form for optimal health and to maintain normal levels of the vitamin.

Even though vitamin D should be supplemented to assist in calcium absorption and to provide other benefits, it is important to note that taking excessively high amounts of vitamin D supplements can cause adverse effects, a condition known as vitamin D toxicity. Vitamin D toxicity has been linked to symptoms such as hypercalcemia, nausea, vomiting, diarrhea, constipation, and weakness.

Exogenous Ketone Supplements

The very first exogenous ketone supplement was released to the world in 2014. Since this time, many new exogenous ketone supplements have been released on the market. There are mixed opinions regarding these supplements, both positive and negative. While these supplements have positive effects to the ketogenic lifestyle, their long-term effects are not known yet. Even though there are currently studies being conducted to find if these supplements may yield negative effects in the body over a longer term, it is still too soon to provide effective results.

Remember that it can be a slow and difficult transition getting the body to go from sugar-burning to fat-burning (ketosis). Some people suffer from keto flu during this transition. So, the aim of exogenous ketone supplements is to bridge the gap and make this transition to enter ketosis faster. The purpose of exogenous ketone supplements is to provide energy and to possibly decrease cravings.

To understand the composition of exogenous ketone supplements, we first must consider ketones in general. The three primary types of ketones include acetone ketones, acetoacetate ketones, and beta-hydroxybutyric acid. Beta-hydroxybutyric acid is often simply referred to as BHB or 3-hydroxybutyrate.

Furthermore, ketones can be classified into two broad categories, endogenous and exogenous ketones. Endog-enous ketones refer to ketones that are produced internally in a person's body. Exogenous ketones refer to ketones that are not produced internally but rather extracted from an external source. This is the type of ketones in the form of ketone supplements.

The majority of supplements that are promoted as exogenous ketone supplements contain beta-acid

(BHB). The majority of the BHB ketone is converted into acetoacetic acid.

Exogenous Ketones ≠ Raspberry Ketones

Before we look at the different exogenous ketones supplements, we first want to cover a very important subject. There has been a lot of confusion recently with the term "ketones." While some supplements have claimed to provide "exogenous ketones," there are also many supplements that promote the ingredient "raspberry ketones." Many people have opted for those supplements with the active ingredient "raspberry ketones" since it sounds the same as "exogenous ketones" but costs much less. These "raspberry ketone" supplements also make various claims regarding the effectiveness of their "ketones" for weight loss.

Unfortunately, these two substances are not the same. In fact, they do not share any type of similarities. As explained above, exogenous ketones are actual ketones similar to those that are produced in the human body that are used as an alternate energy source instead of glucose.

Raspberry ketones, on the other hand, are derived from a chemical found in certain plants. Even though called "raspberry" ketones, the chemical is present in many other plants, including rhubarb, pine tree bark, apples, grapes, peaches, and kiwifruit.

These "ketone" supplements only became popular after Dr. Oz mentioned them as a "miracle fat-burner" on his television series. The supplements became popular in 2012, two years prior to the release of the first exogenous ketone supplements.

Even though raspberry ketones became very popular, there is very little evidence that supports their use in aiding a person in burning fat and losing weight faster. Some studies have proven that these chemicals may increase the rate of the user's metabolism a little, but it does not seem like the increase in metabolism is significant enough to provide impressive weight loss results.

The point I am trying to make is that people should avoid opting for raspberry ketones and should be careful not to confuse them with exogenous ketones. The two supplements are completely different. Raspberry ketones will not help a person enter ketosis faster and will not help the body turn to fat as a source of energy. This is something that exogenous ketones will do.

Two Types of Exogenous Ketone Supplements

Now that we have explained the fact that exogenous ketones and raspberry ketones are NOT the same, the next step is to understand the different forms of the exogenous ketone supplements that are currently available. There are two main forms of these supplements—one contains ketones that are derived from natural sources; the other contains ketones that have been synthetically produced in a laboratory. Understanding the difference between these will help you buy a more effective supplement in the end.

Ketone salts—ketone salts, also called BHB mineral salts or ketone mineral salts, are the most popular form of the exogenous ketone supplement. Ketone salts supplements contain natural substances instead of compounds that have been produced in a laboratory. They utilize beta-hydroxybutyrate acid (BHB) as their primary type of ketone. That BHB is then mixed with a sodium solution. Some supplements may contain some calcium or potassium in addition to the sodium to help reduce the user's risk of experiencing the dreaded symptoms of keto flu.

At the moment, all exogenous supplements on the market, except for one, utilize ketone salts in their formula instead of the other type (ketone esters, explained below). Popular ketone salts include Keto OS and KetoForce.

Ketone Esters—the other form of ketone supplements are called ketone esters. This form of ketones is primarily used in research studies. With ketone esters, a ketone body is bound with alcohol. This helps to increase the liver's ability to use the ketone. Ketone esters are known to taste very bad and have only recently become a point of interest among manufacturers of exogenous ketone supplements.

In 2018, a brand known as HVMN developed the world's very first commercially-available exogenous ketone supplement that utilizes ketone esters instead of ketone salts. This marked a significant advancement in the supplements industry and provided a way to deliver ketones to the user that is metabolized and used by their body at a much faster rate as compared to those supplements that use ketone salts.

The Benefits of Exogenous Ketone Supplements

Ketogenic supplements are used for different reasons. The primary reason that's been mentioned already is to help the body enter the ketosis state, which is the ultimate goal of the ketogenic diet, without experiencing as many side effects. The other benefits of taking exogenous ketones include:

- Improvements in physical and sports performance

- Neuroprotective benefits that help to reduce the risk of Parkinson's disease and Alzheimer's disease

- A significant reduction in low-grade chronic inflammation

- Anti-carcinogenic benefits, which can reduce the risk of cancer and improve the survival rate of those who have developed cancer.

Side Effects of Exogenous Ketone Supplements

Even though a person can gain many benefits from using exogenous ketone supplements, there are some drawbacks that need to be considered as well. Similar to how a regular ketogenic diet can cause a person to experience side effects due to an imbalance in electrolyte levels, the same thing can occur when opting for exogenous ketone supplements. This is why a lot of exogenous supplements either advise the user to take additional supplements, or they already include in them certain electrolytes, such as sodium, calcium, potassium, and magnesium.

Some people who use these supplements may also experience halitosis, or bad breath, as a side effect. This is a common side effect when following a ketogenic diet alone. The bad breath is the result of the body starting to metabolize the fat that is present in a person's body instead of using the carbohydrates they eat. Fortunately, when adding exogenous supplements, the bad breath side effect of ketosis tends to clear up much faster as compared to entering ketosis without the use of such supplements.

Another concern that many people also may experience during the first few days after they start to use a supplement that contains either keto salts or keto esters is some gastrointestinal distress. This is not a side effect that everyone will experience, however. Additionally, most people who do experience flatulence as a side effect are the ones who consume excessively high levels of these supplements. This side effect tends to clear up rather quickly as the digestive system simply needs to "get used" to the ketones that the person is taking.

Hypoglycemia is another concern that a lot of people worry about, but usually does not become a problem in the majority of people who uses exogenous ketone supplements. This is because by the time the blood glucose level of the user becomes low, the body would already be able to provide adequate supplies of ketones (as a source of energy) to the brain and other parts of the body. This, in turn, means even when blood glucose levels become low, symptoms associated with hypoglycemia will usually not develop.

Supplements and Keto-Related Nutrition Gaps

Thus far, we have covered supplements that become useful during the transition from a body that relies on carbohydrates and glucose for energy, to a body that rather utilizes fat, which is converted into ketones, for energy (i.e., ketosis).

Now, we want to turn our focus toward supplements that a person can use to avoid nutritional deficiencies while they are following a ketogenic diet. While the diet is beneficial, there are numerous restrictions placed on the foods that a person can eat. In turn, this often makes it very hard for a person to ensure they eat an adequate amount of all vital nutrients that their body relies on daily.

In such cases, supplements can be used to fill these "gaps" in nutrients that are caused by the ketogenic diet. We have already discussed the fact that following this particular type of diet puts a person at risk of suffering a deficiency in important electrolytes, including magnesium, sodium, and potassium. Apart from these deficiencies, there are other nutrients that are sometimes a concern.

The majority of common nutritional deficiencies with this diet can be effectively avoided by simply planning out the meals and foods that will be eaten. Unfortunately, it can sometimes be difficult to get the right combination of foods to ensure a low intake of carbs, moderate intake of protein, and a high intake of fats, while also balancing the intake of all essential nutrients. That's where supplements come in.

Vitamin B Family

B vitamins all play important roles in the human body that make them essential to human health. They are readily available in many foods, but unfortunately a number of these foods are known to be high in carbohydrates. Thus, opting for a multivitamin supple-ment that contains the seven main vitamin B types can help to ensure a person gets enough of these vitamins to support their particular functions.

The seven primary types of vitamin Bs include:

Vitamin B1—this vitamin, also known as thiamin, plays a vital role in the breakdown of proteins, as well as fats and carbohydrates. Thus, vitamin B1 is essential in the ketogenic diet. In addition to its function in assisting with the breakdown of certain nutrients, thiamin is important in the production of energy within the human body. Furthermore, it is known to contribute to the optimal functioning of nerve cells.

Vitamin B2—also known as riboflavin, this is another particularly important B vitamin that is involved in the processing of amino acids. Riboflavin also plays a crucial role in the metabolism and processing of fats in the human body, making this another essential nutrient for people following this diet. Additionally, it contrib-utes to the production of energy from macronutrients and serves as a powerful antioxidant.

Vitamin B3—vitamin B3, more commonly known as niacin, contributes to a lot of functions in the human body. It is known to contribute to healthy skin, as well as to assist with regulating the function of the body's central nervous system. Additionally, niacin is known to assist with the production of sex hormones, including estrogen and testosterone. The vitamin is also crucial for the respiration of cells in the human body.

Vitamin B5—vitamin B5, also known as pantothenic acid, is important for extracting energy from the fats that are present in the human body. This factor makes it a vital part of the ketogenic diet since fats serve as the primary source of energy in the body of a person who follows this diet. Pantothenic acid also contributes to the production of the body's red blood cells. Steroid hormone production greatly relies on the presence of vitamin B5.

Vitamin B6—vitamin B6, also called pyridoxine, is important for the metabolism of carbohydrates. It also serves a purpose in red blood cell production, as well as the formation of important proteins in the body. Furthermore, it has an impact on the well-being of the immune system and affects brain function.

Vitamin B7—vitamin B7, also known as biotin, plays a very important role in the synthesis of fat in the human body. It is also responsible for amino acid synthesis and the metabolism of energy. Healthy levels of biotin in the human body help to maintain a normal level of cholesterol in the blood circulatory system.

Vitamin B9—vitamin B9, or folate as it is commonly known, assists the body in producing red blood cells. These red blood cells, in turn, help to ensure proper oxygen delivery to all tissues within the body. Folate is also a crucial supplement for pregnant women, as it assists with the growth of the fetus, as well as the development of the unborn baby's nervous system.

Vitamin B12—vitamin B12, also called cyanocobalamin, has many functions in the human body, making it one of the most important vitamins to consume. Cyanocobalamin is known to assist with red blood cell formation, as well as provide better mental clarity. One particular reason why B12 is an essential part of a ketogenic diet is that this vitamin is involved in the process where fatty acids are broken down into a form that can be used for the production of energy.

Vitamin B Deficiencies

When a person fails to obtain an adequate supply of B vitamins, they can develop a number of unpleasant symptoms. The most common symptoms associated with vitamin B deficiencies include confusion, paranoia, anger, depression, and anxiety.

Additionally, there are a couple of physiological symptoms that may develop when levels of B vitamins in the human body become low. These may include a tingling sensation in the feet, as well as the hands. Some people may have problems with their ability to walk normally. Heart palpitations may develop. Additionally, many people may find that they develop symptoms that are associated with insomnia. In turn, this may affect their cognitive function during their day-to-day activities.

Omega-3 Fatty Acids

Another important supplement that many people take while they are on the ketogenic diet is omega-3 fatty acids. This is not the most crucial supplement for individuals who include fatty fish in their daily diets— fatty fish is, after all, a great source of healthy fats, which play a particularly important part in this type of diet. For those who do not eat enough fish, using supplements that contain omega-3 fatty acids can be beneficial.

It is recommended to consume approximately 4,000 mg omega-3 fatty acids on a daily basis. This is not the daily intake recommendation for the ketogenic diet specifically but is a general recommendation regardless of a person's diet.

Omega-3 fatty acids play many roles in the human body. Adequate supplementation of these fatty acids can provide numerous benefits as well, such as:

- Improvements in cardiovascular well-being, which, in turn, reduces the risk of heart disease

- Improvements in the blood circulatory system's ability to transport oxygen throughout the body

- A reduction in blood pressure levels should a person struggle with hypertension, as well as the regulation of normal blood pressure levels

These fatty acids are also known to help reduce inflammation in the body. Furthermore, omega-3 fatty acids are crucial to the development of the brain. In older individuals, these compounds play a vital role in maintaining a healthy brain, as well as in reducing the risk of certain diseases, such as Alzheimer's disease.

Omega-3 fatty acids are readily available in when you consume fatty fish, such as albacore tuna, mackerel, and sardines. They are also found in various non-fish foods, such as egg yolks, chia seeds, walnuts, hemp seeds, and soybean oil. For those who are unable to properly fit in an adequate amount of food to supplement their bodies with omega-3 fatty acids, the use of fish oil tablets or krill oil tablets can be a great way to ensure a daily intake of 4,000 mg of omega-3.

While the intake of these fatty acids should play an important part of a ketogenic diet, whether it is through food sources or with the use of supplements, individuals should avoid taking in too much of them. It is not yet completely clear what the side effects of excessive omega-3 intake may be, but one report did note that it can cause problems with the immune system. In particular, the study pointed out that high levels of omega-3 can make the immune system less capable in fighting against bacteria and other pathogenic microorganisms that enter the body.

Vitamin C

Vitamin C is probably the most popular vitamin in the entire world. It is the go-to vitamin for people who catch a cold or develop the flu. This vitamin is known to be a very powerful antioxidant and plays a crucial role in the maintenance of a healthy immune system. Additionally, vitamin C helps to prevent the accumulation of LDL cholesterol, often referred to as bad cholesterol. By reducing the buildup of LDL cholesterol, vitamin C further helps to improve health.

There are many other ways that vitamin C contributes to a healthy body. For example, it is important in the production of collagen. Collagen is a substance that helps to keep blood vessels strong and is also essential in the maintenance of strong muscles.

Citrus fruits, such as oranges, contain large amounts of carbohydrates but are also known as the primary sources of vitamin C. This can make it more difficult to obtain an adequate supply of vitamin C while following a ketogenic diet. There are, luckily, many other foods that contain vitamin C. These include cauliflower, kale, broccoli, and spinach.

Additionally, vitamin C supplements are readily available on the shelves of pharmacies, as well as most grocery stores and supermarkets. These supplements are also cheap.

The daily recommended intake for vitamin C is between 65 mg and 90 mg, but a person can safely consume up to 2,000mg of this vitamin on a daily basis without experiencing side effects.

Even though side effects are very uncommon with the use of vitamin C, individuals should note that extremely high doses of the vitamin can cause them to experience some adverse reactions. These may include abdominal cramping, diarrhea, sleeping difficulties, nausea and vomiting, heartburn, and headaches.

Iron

While the ketogenic diet does not put a person at a particularly higher risk of suffering an iron deficiency, it is important to take note of the foods included in your diet and ensure that there is an adequate supply of iron. Iron plays crucial roles in the body, and it can become harmful when its levels fall too low.

Iron is essential in the formation of hemoglobin. Without hemoglobin, the body is unable to transfer oxygen from the lungs to the rest of their body. Additionally, iron is also important in the metabolism of energy, it helps to stimulate improvements in brain function, and it plays a role in healthy muscle function.

Foods that are high in iron and also perfect for those following a ketogenic diet include eggs, meat, dark chocolate, broccoli, spinach, and pumpkin seeds. Iron supplements can help to increase the intake of this nutrient in case the foods in a person's diet do not make up for the recommended daily dosage.

Individuals should consume between 8 mg and 30 mg of iron on a daily basis. It is important to stay within this guideline as too much iron can lead to a condition known as iron poisoning.

Iron poisoning can be fatal, especially when excessively high levels of iron are consumed in a short period of time. Symptoms usually start with abdominal pain and nausea, often followed by vomiting. Other symptoms may include breathing difficulty, fluid accumulation in the lungs, headaches, fever, dizziness, low blood pressure, weak pulse, and even seizures. Symptoms that are linked to jaundice may also develop as the high iron levels may cause damage to the liver.

Green Powders for Optimal Nutritional Intake

Thousands of people who follow a ketogenic diet have noticed the benefits of using one single product that can help fill common "gaps" in their nutrition: "green powders." These green powders usually eliminate the need for multivitamin supplements and other types of supplements often used to increase the intake of vitamins, minerals, and other compounds. This is because the powders usually include the perfect blend of vegetable and plant extracts to provide optimal levels of nutrients.

There are quite a large variety of green powder products on the market, but when opting for this type of nutritional supplement while on a ketogenic diet, it is essential to look for options that are promoted specifically for the keto diet. The "keto" options usually consist of a great nutrient combination, but without containing the carbohydrates that a person would usually also consume should they opt for the vegetables that are used in the product in their "whole food" state.

Opt for green powders that contain no filler ingredients, but rather only pure plant extracts. This ensures maximum benefits without your wasting money or exposing your body to unpleasant toxins and harmful substances. It is also a good idea to opt for one of the "power green powder supplements" that have organic ingredients in them, as compared to those with non-organic ingredients.

Some of these products may include additional ingredients that are also focused specifically on the ketogenic diet. This often includes MCT oil powder, for example.

MCT Supplements and Keto

The majority of people interested in a ketogenic diet will find in their research on it the term "MCT" mentioned somewhere. MCT means "medium-chain triglycerides." This is a type of healthy fat. Apart from medium-chain fats, there are also long-chain fats and short-chain fats. Many people describe the "short," "medium," or "long" terms to be like "handles" that are attached to the fats. A shorter "chain" means the fat is easier for the body to break down and use as a source of energy.

Medium-chain triglycerides are often considered the perfect quick source of energy for people following a ketogenic diet. This is because the medium-chain fats are easily broken down by the human body and, in turn, can be used for energy at a relatively fast rate.

MCT fats are popular because they are easy to digest and they have also been scientifically proven to help increase the production of ketones in the body. Furthermore, they are also considered a "clean" energy source. For many people, these fats play a crucial role in their ketogenic diet.

MCT supplements can be used when starting out on this type of diet, as they will help the body switch faster to utilizing fat for energy. When ketones are produced faster, the body may also adapt to the use of ketones (over glucose) as its energy source at a faster rate, leading to a significant reduction in the symptoms experienced during the potential "keto flu" phase.

The primary source of medium-chain triglycerides is coconut oil. In fact, more than 60% of the fats that are found in coconut oil are considered to be medium-chain fats. This makes coconut oil an important source of these fats for people who are implementing a ketogenic diet.

Other sources of medium-chain fats include cheese, milk, yogurt, and butter.

MCT oil and MCT oil powder are often classified under their own category of ketone supplements: ketone oils. This is because this particular supplement works so great in boosting the production of ketones in the human body.

MCT supplements are available in different forms. While it is possible to turn to coconut oil to increase the intake of medium-chain fats, many people find that the use of specific MCT supplements works better. Most commonly, these individuals would either opt for MCT oil or, alternatively, for MCT oil powder. Both are great sources of these fats to be used for boosting the body's ability to produce ketones quickly and more effectively.

Each of these supplement types is used in its own way. Individuals who opt for MCT oil can use the oil as an alternative to coconut oil or any other type of cooking oil. It has the added benefit of not causing food to have a coconut flavor when cooking. Additionally, the oil can be used to make a salad dressing. Note that since the oil does not have a flavor, it would be a good idea to mix it with other ingredients, such as a few herbs, to add a taste to the dressing.

Some people also add MCT oil to their smoothies. This is a great way to suppress appetite, and most people find that it helps them stay full for a longer period of time. Since the oil does not have a distinct flavor, it can also be used in tea and coffee.

A lot of people do prefer the MCT oil powder instead of the oil, however. There are a few reasons why the powder is a preferred option. Firstly, it is known that MCT oil powder causes fewer side effects (discussed below) when you first introduce it in your diet as compared to pure MCT oil. The powder is also considered a more convenient option for mixing with coffee and other beverages, as well as to sprinkle over food. The powder does not present any taste, so it will not affect the flavor of the food it is added to.

Benefits of MCT Oil Supplements

There are four particular reasons why many people opt for the inclusion of MCT oil supplements in their ketogenic diet. These include:

- The medium-chain fats have been proven to provide a significant improvement in a person's ability to lose weight fast. It has a type of thermogenic effect in the body, which speeds up the metabolism.

- People who use MCT oil supplements usually experience significant improvements in their energy levels. This can be great to get over any fatigue during the first week of ketosis and can also provide sustainable energy for those who are already well on their way with a ketogenic diet. The medium-chain fats are quickly converted into energy.

- MCT oil supplements have an antibacterial effect in the body, which helps to reduce the presence of parasites, bacteria, and other pathogenic microorganisms that may be present in the gastrointestinal tract.

- The fact that MCT oil also acts as an antioxidant in the body helps to reduce inflammation, boost heart health, improve brain function, and contributes to an overall healthier body.

Side Effects of MCT Oil Supplements

While the benefits of these supplements often get the spotlight when people talk about them and their ability to improve the experience of the ketogenic diet, it is important to note that some people may experience certain side effects while using MCT oil supplements as well. Fortunately, the majority of side effects are mild and usually do not pose a health threat. Furthermore, the side effects most often clear up within a few days as the body gets used to the new supplement.

The side effects that may develop when a person starts to use supplements that contain MCT oil include irritability, stomach discomfort, diarrhea, nausea, vomiting, and intestinal gas.

In some cases, a person may also develop a deficiency in essential fatty acids. This usually only occurs when the person consumes an excessively large amount of MCT oil supplements. For this reason, it is highly recommended to avoid taking more than the advised daily dosage, which can usually be found on the container of the product purchased (each product contains a different composition of medium-chat fats, which means they will have unique dosage instructions).

Apart from being aware of these possible side effects, individuals interested in using MCT oil supplements should note that these medium-chat fats can have adverse reactions among people with certain diseases. In particular, those who have been previously diagnosed with diabetes are not advised to take supplements that contain these fats. Furthermore, MCT oil supplements have been deemed potentially dangerous for individuals with liver disease, especially those with cirrhosis.

Energy Maintenance Supplements and Keto

For many people, the ketogenic diet is a great way to gain a significant boost in their energy levels. During the early stages, however, it may be difficult as energy levels may first become lower before they are boosted. Fortunately, there are certain supplements that may be helpful in boosting energy and stamina. Different types of supplements have been suggested for various pur-poses. Let's take a look at the most popular ones.

Green tea supplements—green tea is naturally rich in caffeine, but the caffeine found in these supplements usually does not have the same effect like that of coffee, for example. While still a stimulant, people often feel less jittery when they opt for caffeine found in green tea. While these supplements may not be particularly useful in boosting a person's physical performance, they are good options for boosting mental performance. Most people find that using these supplements helps them experience improvements in their mental alertness specifically. It is not necessary to only opt for supple-ments that contain green tea extracts; simply making a cup of green tea can also be a good option.

Chlorella supplements—some people have also found the use of chlorella supplements to be a good option for helping them maintain optimal levels of energy during the day. Chlorella is a natural plant extract. It is known to be highly effective in reducing the risk of experiencing fatigue when the body first enters ketosis. Once in ketosis, the supplement can be great for ensuring energy levels do not deplete during the day.

The ingredient of interest in these supplements is known as chlorella growth factor. This substance contains both DNA and RNA compounds that have been scientifically proven to make the transportation of energy between various cells in the human body more effective. While the most popular way to increase the intake of chlorella growth factor is through the use of the capsules, the supplement is also available in the form of a powder. The powder can easily be added to a smoothie, or even just added to some water. Some people also find that sprinkling some of the powder over their food helps to increase their intake of this supplement without extra effort.

"Keto-Friendly" Workout Supplements

Exercising is an important part of any diet, be it the ketogenic diet or any other type of diet. Many people who adopt this particular diet still want to build muscles and continue to work out at the gym, but they would not be able to continue opting for the standard supplements that are often used pre-and post-workout (because the standard ones contain too many carbohydrates). For this reason, it is important to also look at workout supplements that are good for people following a ketogenic diet. Below, I share some pre-and post-workout supplements that provide the perfect way to perform well at the gym and experience optimal muscle growth and recovery after the workout is done.

Creatine monohydrate—this is a relatively popular supplement that is used by quite a large number of athletes and individuals who are trying to build more muscle mass. Various scientific studies have proven the effectiveness of this supplement. Creatine monohydrate can help to increase the overall physical performance of a person while they are participating in exercise. Additionally, the supplement can also increase physical strength and potentially help to increase the rate at which muscle mass develops.

Branched chain amino acids—branched chain amino acid supplements, often promoted as BCAAs, are important in the process of building muscle mass during physical activity. In addition to being useful in building muscle mass faster, BCAAs may also help to maintain existing muscle mass. Various scientific studies have proven the effectiveness of this supplement. BCAAs can increase physical strength and potentially also help to increase the rate at which muscle mass develops.

L-Glutamine—another great supplement for those individuals who are following a ketogenic diet and require an effective post-workout supplement is L-glutamine. During intense workout protocols, reserves of glutamine in the body quickly reduce. Glutamine contributes to faster and better recovery post-workout. Thus, by supplementing the body with L-glutamine, recovery time after a workout session can be reduced. This may also help to reduce soreness.

L-glutamine is also a powerful antioxidant that helps to protect the body at a cellular level against free radical damage. Thus, when levels of glutamine are reduced during exercise, it also means that the compound cannot effectively protect cells in the body. This makes it is even more important to supplement the body with L-glutamine. In those individuals following a standard diet, L-glutamine is usually obtained from food sources, but many of the foods that contain this antioxidant are high in carbohydrates, which makes them difficult to include in a ketogenic diet.

This supplement is often taken before a workout starts to reduce the effect that exercise will have on the naturally stored levels of glutamine in the body. The supplement can be obtained by taking capsules or by using a powdered supplement.

In summary, because the ketogenic diet puts your body into ketosis and also entails eating primarily healthy fats, many people opt to do cleanses when getting started, taking supplements when getting started, and taking supplements regularly throughout. Because your body needs to reorient itself when it changes from sugar-burning to fat-burning (ketosis), doing a cleanse beforehand and taking supplements during your start of the diet can be a great idea. To get any nutrients that might be falling through the gap, you might want to take supplements regularly as part of your keto lifestyle. Use the information in this chapter to decide what makes most sense for you, and consider getting advice from your doctor or a nutritionist as well. And remember, a great source for your supplements is my site www.loveyournewyou.com. Put in the promo code BOOK at www.loveyournewyou.com/book at checkout, so you, as a reader of my book, can enjoy a discount.

We ended this chapter by looking at how certain supplements can assist you when doing exercise while on a ketogenic diet. The next chapter focuses on exercise, so you can get educated on the role of fitness, working out, and exercise in the keto lifestyle.

Amber S.'s Message

Amber, a 21-year-old female, started the ketogenic lifestyle and, 8 months in, she has lost 60 pounds. Her self esteem has greatly improved, and now she is feeling confident and wanting to go back to school, something that wasn't on her agenda 8 months ago. April 2018

References

https://www.nutraceuticalsworld.com/contents/ view_online-exclusives/2016-10-31/over-170-million-americans-take-dietary-supplements/

https://www.medicalnewstoday.com/articles/ 319196.php

https://www.epilepsysociety.org.uk/ketogenic-diet#.W2MzeNJMTIU

https://ods.od.nih.gov/factsheets/Magnesium-healthProfessional/

https://www.webmd.com/vitamins/ai/ingredientmono-1262/raspberry-ketone

https://today.oregonstate.edu/archives/2013/oct/excess-omega-3-fatty-acids-could-lead-negative-health-effects

https://www.mayoclinic.org/healthy-lifestyle/nutrition-and-healthy-eating/expert-answers/vitamin-c/faq-20058030

https://www.healthline.com/health/iron-poisoning#symptoms

https://drjockers.com/5-reasons-use-mct-oil-ketosis/

https://www.webmd.com/vitamins/ai/ingredientmono-915/medium-chain-triglycerides-mcts

https://www.sciencedaily.com/releases/2017/02/170223124259.htm

When you feel like quitting, think about why you started.

—Anonymous

Chapter 8
Exercise and Keto

Out of all my patients who have started this new lifestyle, only a handful began exercising as the same time as starting the ketogenic diet. While I don't have a problem with anyone exercising right away, many get overwhelmed by changing their diet and adding exercise. That's OK—you will still see benefits if you don't exercise right away.

Often once my patients start seeing significant weight loss, feeling better, and having more energy in the first 1 to 2 months, they bring up exercise—asking what they should do and how often. In 1 Corinthians 9:24–25 it says, "Don't you realize that in a race everyone runs, but only one person gets the prize? So run to win! All athletes are disciplined in their training. They do it to win a prize that will fade away, but we do it for an eternal prize." In this race that we have here on Earth against weight gain and being unhealthy, I encourage you to keep running and keep your focus on the prize that you seek. But honor Him and don't forget the main prize.

When a person combines exercise with a ketogenic diet, the body can burn more fat. Your body needs an energy source. When you get to a point where you are burning ketones for energy instead of sugar—what is called "ketosis"—more fat can be burned. The ketones are utilized instead of sugar for your body's energy source.

Let's look at some different types of athletes and their bodies. You, like me, probably will never look like these guys. But I want to point out how they train and the results of their training. Comparing a sprinter versus a marathoner, you can see some differences. The sprinter is usually very muscular and lean. The marathoner is usually skinny. Why is that? It's because of their process. A sprinter and marathoner do both short, quick bursts of training and long-distance type training. The difference is what they do the most: short, quick distance for the sprinter and longer steady training for the marathoner. As far as weight training, both lift weights. But the sprinter does more heavy lifting, and the marathoner does more light lifting. Neither training is wrong but how you train will determine your body style. As I discuss different types of exercise later, keep in mind the type of body you are looking to get.

What I recommend depends on where you're at. If you haven't done any exercise in the recent past, then simply walking is a good start.

If you have some background with exercising and are able to do it, then you can progress to more intense type of activities. Check out my website for more in-depth information on this topic: www.ourketogeniclife.com.

If you have been exercising and you start a ketogenic lifestyle, the first 1 to 2 weeks will be an adjustment period. Remember that you are switching energy sources. So in the first weeks, you may notice a decrease in stamina. This will not last. In fact, after a few weeks, you will probably see an increase in energy. Just be aware and stay the course.

Types of Exercise

Extended Walks—doing a steady type of exercise is not the best way to burn fat. However, if you haven't been used to exercise, this is a great place to start. Instead of just sitting on the couch watching TV, start the process of changing your mindset.

Once or twice a week, walk for 30 minutes. Not at a grandma's pace, but also not at a sprinter's pace. To determine your pace, make sure you are a little short of breath to where you couldn't carry on a normal conversation. This is a good place to start and also a good type of exercise to sprinkle in with the following exercise types.

High intensity interval training (HIIT)—this program is something that can be done at home, outside, or in a weight room. First, pick an exercise, such as a sprint. Then exercise for 10 minutes following this pattern: warm up for a minute or two, complete the exercise you picked for 30 seconds, then walk for 60 seconds, continue to alternate back and forth between the sprinting for 30 seconds and walking for 60 seconds. As you progress, increase the total exercise time. Some examples of great HIIT exercises include run/walk, jump rope, bicycle, elliptical, and burpees.

Tabata—this is a 4-minute routine easily done anywhere. Go online and find a free Tabata timer. Next select an exercise, such as a push-up. Click "start" on your timer. You will do your chosen exercise for 20 seconds, then rest for 10 seconds. You will alternate this 8 times, which will take 4 minutes total. Then pick a different exercise and do this again. Pick 2 or 3 different exercises each day.

Some examples of great Tabata exercises include push-ups, burpees, jump rope, pull-ups, step-ups, planks, body weight squats, mountain climbers, jumping jacks, sprints, and stationary bike riding.

Weight training—whether you go to the weight room or start a program at home, increasing your strength and muscle mass will not only increase weight loss, but also help prevent future medical conditions. You will feel better, which will only motivate you to continue the process. This doesn't have to be difficult or intimidating.

Start with a full body workout targeting one exercise per body part. Do one exercise 10 times, and 3 sets total of that exercise. For example, if you are doing a dumbbell chest press, pick a weight, lie down, and do 10 reps. Wait 30 to 60 seconds (this is your short rest time) and then do another 10 reps. Wait again and do a final 10 reps (that's 3 sets total). Then move onto the next exercise.

Here is sample routine that uses dumbbells (DB) and your body:

- Lying DB chest press—works your chest

- Bent-over DB row—works your back

- DB shoulder press—works your shoulders

- DB overhead triceps extension—works your triceps

- DB biceps curl—works your biceps

- Step-ups on a bench with or without DB—works your quads

- DB bent-over Romanian—works your hamstrings

- Plank on your elbows—works your abdomen muscle, holding as long as possible

Let me add that if you don't know how to do any of the exercises I listed or don't know where the exact muscles are located in the body that an exercise works, do an internet search and you'll find explanations. For instance, search the phrase "DB shoulder press," and you'll find many options of people demonstrating it on videos. Search the term "hamstrings," and you'll find charts that show you where in the body the hamstrings are.

I urge you to check out www.ourketogeniclife.com to get further suggestions on exercise routines, especially because you will need to change your routines up over time. The types of exercises I've given in this chapter—extended walks, HIIT, Tabata, and weight training—are a great starting point. Doing any of them 2 to 3 times per week will offer your body and mind tremendous benefits, and it will propel your weight loss.

In addition to introducing exercise to your ketogenic lifestyle, another great way to accelerate weight loss and improve the overall health of your body is to introduce intermittent fasting. I know—some of you are probably concerned or even frightened of the idea of fasting. You might think it's very painful and dangerous. In the next chapter, I'm going to dispel those myths. You are going to learn multiple safe and healthy techniques for fasting for select blocks of time. As a matter of fact, after reading the chapter, I predict you'll be eager to start your first fast!

Clark H's Statistics

Clark had heart disease and thyroid problems, and he struggled to lose weight. He tried other solutions to improve his health and lose weight in the past, but nothing stuck. Either he found difficulty sticking to it, or he quit when he didn't see the improvements he was looking for. On October 8, 2017, Clark weighed 239. Now in April of 2018, he weighs 200. He feels better and has more energy. How did Clark lose 39 pounds? He began a consistent walking routine. Now he is expanding his exercise program—doing HIIT and Tabata workouts too. Clark's body thanks him!

The best of all medicines is resting and fasting.

—Ben Franklin

Chapter 9
Intermittent Fasting

In this chapter, you will learn all things intermittent fasting. We'll start by going over what it is—and what it's not. From there, we'll explore its health benefits, including weight loss as well as other improvements. After that, you'll be presented with six different types of intermittent fasts as well as my recommendations for getting started with intermittent fasting. Finally, I'll share some helpful resources, apps, and other tools, so you have even more support when you incorporate this powerful practice into your life. As you'll soon learn, intermittent fasting combined with a ketogenic lifestyle sets you up for optimal health, both in terms of weight loss but also on the cellular level.

What It Is and Isn't

Let us start by taking a look at what intermittent fasting is. The term has become quite popular in recent years, but there is still a lot of confusion in regards to what it really means and involves. Many people think that the term "intermittent fasting" refers to a diet, but it is not actually a diet. Instead, it is an eating pattern or an eating schedule that people adopt that gives guidance on *when* to eat and *when* not to eat.

To best understand it, let me give you an example of a type of intermittent fast. (I'm explaining it very briefly here, but later in the chapter you'll find an extensive explanation of this type of intermittent fast as well as others.) To understand how intermittent fasting works, let's look at the 16/8 intermittent fast. In the 16/8 fast, you determine an 8-hour block in your day during which you'll eat your meals, and the rest of the hours of the day, 16, is when no eating will occur. For example, you might choose to have your meals sometime between noon and 8 PM (that's the 8-hour block), and you wouldn't eat from 8 PM to noon (that's 16 hours). In doing this, you are fasting for 16 hours, but once those 16 hours end, you eat again.

What's so great about doing this? We'll go into the benefits more extensively later in the chapter, but here's the general idea. By allowing a 16-hour block of time in which no eating occurs, the digestive system is given a break from processing and digesting food continuously, and also insulin levels are lowered. This break is very helpful for the body's overall health. And, this break allows for weight loss.

There are a lot of people who are scared of adopting intermittent fasting because they think that they will starve themselves. This, however, is a myth that holds no truth. Remember, intermittent fasting isn't about calorie restricting. It's simply about scheduling when you eat and when you don't eat. During the window of time when you will be eating your meals, you aren't required to restrict calories. However, during the block of time in which no eating occurs, no eating occurs. That's when you are giving your body and digestive system a break.

An important fact that you should know when it comes to discussing this method of eating is that since it is not classified as a diet, it does not decide the types of food that you will be eating. It is up to you to decide what you want to eat. A healthy, balanced diet that is filled with foods high in essential nutrients will, of course, result in more benefits as compared to stuffing yourself with hamburgers and pizza as soon as the clock strikes 5 PM (or whatever time your eating cycle starts). When opting for fast foods and other food options that are very high in carbohydrates, weight loss may not be a particular benefit that you experience when following this eating pattern.

Because this book is dedicated to the ketogenic lifestyle, you should already know that I highly recommend that you combine intermittent fasting with the ketogenic diet. What this means is that when your eating cycle begins, you choose foods that adhere to the ketogenic diet, which we discussed in depth in previous chapters.

As explained, intermittent fasting involves cycles of eating and abstaining from food. There are different techniques and methods that have been introduced over the last few years, so not everyone will follow this technique in the same way. Generally, however, all options involve periods of time when food is consumed, and then periods when the person completely avoids eating any type of food. Later in this chapter, I'll give you a variety of options for incorporating intermittent fasting into your life in a safe and effective way. Before we look at those particulars, let's find out the myriad health benefits intermittent fasting offers.

The Benefits

There are many different reasons why people use the intermittent fasting technique. Some of these techniques date back to ancient times. For example, in older times, when a village only had a limited food supply, people in the village would often implement a type of fasting technique to help make the food last longer. Careful planning had to go into such a technique as the villagers had to eat enough food to support their bodily functions, at the right times, while still ensuring the inventory of available food could last until more food became available.

Certain religions also have certain celebrations and festivals where people fast. Religions that incorporate fasting include Buddhism, Judaism, Islam, Hinduism,

Bahai, Jainism, Raelism, and Sikhism. Certain types of Christian religions also use fasting for various purposes. This includes Catholicism, Orthodoxy, Mormonism, and Protestantism. These religions use fasting in different ways, and the technique serves a different purpose in each religion. Some religions also only utilize parts of these fasting techniques and will not completely eliminate all foods from a person's diet for a set period of time.

Many people also tend to go on a fast when they feel sick, whether they have contracted the flu or another type of disease. This is because food does not work well with nausea and vomiting, nor with other types of gastrointestinal symptoms.

In modern times, however, more and more people are starting to adopt an intermittent fasting lifestyle. Often it is not because they are sick or because of religious requirements, but rather due to the health benefits that have been associated with this practice of scheduled eating.

Weight Loss Benefits

Intermittent fasting has two particular benefits that should be considered when it comes to losing weight. Firstly, it has been scientifically proven to help shed excess fat. This is a major advantage to opting for this eating pattern. Most programs, diets, and even pills that can be taken to initiate weight loss tend to reduce weight through a reduction in "water weight." Rarely do they truly help a person lose actual fat. With intermittent fasting, however, science has proven that a person burns fat, and their body fat percentage becomes reduced when they implement this technique and strictly stick to the particular eating schedule they have decided on.

The other major benefit in regards to weight loss is that this scheduled eating plan has also been proven to preserve the lean muscle mass in a person's body while they lose weight. This is an important factor that needs to be taken into account. Lean muscle mass is important for several functions of the human body and also helps to make movement more comfortable.

For example, lean muscle mass has been proven beneficial in the prevention of insulin resistance, as well as diabetes. A loss of lean muscle mass has also been associated with a higher incidence of illness. Cancer patients, for example, who lose muscle mass while undergoing treatment are less likely to survive and more likely to experience a recurrence of the disease should they survive, as compared to those who maintain healthier levels of muscle mass.

Furthermore, research has also proven that lean muscle mass helps to maintain stronger bones. When bones are kept in a healthy and strong state, then a person is less likely to experience problems like fragile bones and balance issues. The person will also be less likely to suffer an injury during physical activity. The risk of osteoarthritis and similar diseases are also lower among individuals with stronger bones and better levels of lean muscle mass.

Several suggestions have been made regarding the way that intermittent fasting helps a person lose excess fat while also preserving their existing muscle mass. The effect that these scheduled eating habits have on the body's metabolism is thought to play a significant role here. For example, one research study found that the gut flora, also called the microbiome, is positively affected by intermittent fasting. This, in turn, can help to improve metabolism and make the digestive system more efficient.

Even More Benefits

While weight loss is the most popular reason that people opt for intermittent fasting, it is important to realize that there are <u>more benefits</u> as well. In particular, it has been found that this technique actually changes for the better certain cells in the body. This, in turn, can cause positive changes in human growth hormone regulation, insulin regulation, and even improve the body's ability to repair cells.

Fasting has also been linked to reductions in low-grade chronic inflammation throughout the body, lower levels of oxidative stress in body tissues and cells, as well as potential improvements in a person's cardiovascular health. In turn, this combination of powerful benefits may lead to a longer lifespan. Note: while this has not been proven yet, long-term studies are currently being conducted to see whether these benefits can, in fact, prolong a person's life.

A Harvard Medical School study on intermittent fasting provided evidence that mitochondria of the body's cells get manipulated in a beneficial way among individuals following an intermittent fasting plan. This the study suggested that such an effect in the human body could possibly lead to longer life. It would essentially help the person to age in a healthier way and maintain a healthier overall well-being.

Even though it has been suggested that brain fog might be a side effect of intermittent fasting, one study has suggested that the use of this technique in a person's life on a regular basis may have neuroprotective benefits on their brain—meaning it could help the brain. In particular, they found that this type of lifestyle may help to significantly reduce a person's risk of developing diseases such as Parkinson's and Alzheimer's.

Inflammation has been suggested as the underlying cause of all diseases and illnesses that people experience today. Chronic inflammation often goes unnoticed and only becomes a concern once a person is diagnosed with irritable bowel syndrome, cancer, or another type of disease that the inflammation has contributed to. A University of Illinois study found that intermittent fasting seems to produce anti-inflammatory effects in the human body. These effects have been reported to be more significant and effective among individuals who implement a steady schedule for their fasting windows and who stick to the schedule.

Several studies have suggested that diabetes and insulin resistance may be prevented with intermittent fasting. In particular, a University of Southern California study found that fasting helps to stimulate the production of new cells in the pancreas, which then replace old ones that have been damaged. When such a series of events occur in the body of a person who already has diabetes, the way their body deals with insulin may be improved, due to a better functioning pancreas.

Side Effects of Intermittent Fasting

While there are many benefits to be gained from implementing intermittent fasting into your life, some side effects may also occur. It is important that you know about these, especially if you are currently suffering from a particular medical condition.

When starting intermittent fasting, people sometimes find that the most unpleasant side effects include tiredness, low energy, and hunger. These are all normal effects due to the sudden change in your eating pattern in that you are no longer continuously feeding your body, but instead giving your digestive system a break now and then. Some of the intermittent fasting plans, especially those that require 24-hour periods of fasting, are tougher and will cause more significant side effects. Fortunately, these side effects tend to clear up as your body gets used to this new routine. Keep on schedule to help your body better adapt.

Apart from the low energy and perhaps feelings of hunger, other side effects may also occur. This often includes discomfort when eating because you have gone without food for some time. Also you might eat more than usual once your eating window begins. In turn, this can make your stomach feel excessively full and cause you discomfort.

Another particular problem with intermittent fasting is the fact that many people become hooked on coffee. This is especially a problem during the early phases. They start to feel tired and hungry, so they grab a coffee. As long as it is black coffee and contains no calories (from sugar or milk), it doesn't count as interrupting the fast. While there are certainly benefits to drinking coffee, too much caffeine can become disruptive during sleep, as well as cause anxiety symptoms to develop.

During the fast windows, many people may also find that their athletic and physical performance tends to suffer. It is usually possible to perform certain types of activities of moderate intensity, but heavier regimens are often too difficult. You may not have enough energy to perform those activities.

Other side effects that should be noted include brain fog, diarrhea, headaches, and heartburn.

Different Methods of Intermittent Fasting

To help you get a better idea of how different types of intermittent fasting techniques work and to give you an opportunity to select the one that will work best for you, we will take a look at five of the most common options that people tend to opt for. You'll notice that no matter the type of intermittent fasting, all involve sustained blocks of time in which eating is allowed and dedicated and sustained blocks of time for fasting.

The 16/8 Plan

The 16/8 plan is the most popular method of intermittent fasting. Most intermittent fasters follow this plan. The 16/8 plan is relatively simple to follow and easy to track. You would basically have 16 hours per day when you fast, and 8 hours when you eat. The period of time during which you are allowed to eat, in this case for those 8 hours, is often referred to as the eating window.

All meals that will be consumed in a single day would happen within this 8-hour eating window. Multiple meals can be consumed within these 8 hours, perhaps 2 or 3 meals. Once the 8 hours have passed, however, you would go back into a fasting window and not be allowed to eat anything for the next 16 hours. For instance, you might decide that your eating window is from 12AM to 8 PM (8 hours total), so your fasting window is from 8 PM to 12 AM (16 hours). You might choose your eating window to be from 8AM to 4 PM and your fasting window from 4 PM to 8 AM.

The 16/8 plan is the simplest option for newcomers. Meals can be divided into the 8-hour window, for example, you could have your first meal of the day at 12 AM, the second meal at 5 PM and the third meal at 8 PM. After the final meal, which you eat at 8PM, you would then fast until 12 AM the next day.

To ease your way into the 16/8 plan, some people start with a 14/10 plan, meaning they have a fasting window of 14 hours and an eating window of 10 hours. Over time, once they are comfortable and successful with this, they might change to the 16/8 plan.

The 5/2 Plan

The eat-fast cycle in this plan works throughout the seven days of the week (as opposed to hours within a 24-hour period). Five days make up the eating window, and two days the fasting window.

Individuals who adopt the 5/2 plan, often referred to as the "fast diet," would need to dedicate two "fasting" days each week during which they will significantly restrict their caloric intake for the entire day. It is recommended to choose two days that are not consecutive. For example, you could choose to fast on Tuesdays and Thursdays, or Tuesdays and Fridays.

During the 5 days that count as the eating window, you eat like you normally do and you do not have to place restrictions on your caloric intake (although, a healthy diet would be best!). On the two days that have been dedicated to fasting, you restrict your intake of calories to either 500 or 600 for the entire day. Women should restrict their caloric intake to 500 calories while men are allowed to go up to 600 calories. Most people decide to get those few calories in two small, low-calorie meals on the two fast days. For example, women may consume two meals that have 250 calories each. Men might eat two 300-calorie meals.

The Alternative-Day Plan

This is a more advanced-type of intermittent fasting plan that is not followed by as many people. As the name suggests, you would be alternating between your days as a cycle. One day would be your eating window, and the next day would be a fasting day, and so on.

This particular plan has been split into different sub-categories, but they have very similar features. Some require you to completely avoid eating on your fast days, while others suggest eating some foods on fasting days, but not to exceed around 500 calories during the entire fast day.

The main reason why many people do not opt for this plan is that they would essentially have to get in bed hungry on the fast days, which can make it difficult to fall asleep. This plan is also more likely to make a person feel hungry as compared to the 16/8 plan, for example. If you hope to do this alternate-day intermittent fasting plan, a good idea is to start fasting following another plan and then gradually move to this one. This makes the transitioning phase much more bearable.

The Eat-Stop-Eat Method

This method has become very popular recently but is often not recommended for individuals who are new to intermittent fasting. It can be difficult to adopt the eat-stop-eat method, which is why it is usually advised to start with the 16/8 plan and then to gradually move up until you can reach the fast window for this option. This option does not, however, include a fasting period every day.

For the the eat-stop-eat method you need to choose one or two days every week, which will be your fast days. During these days, you abstain from eating any solid foods for a period of 24 hours in total. It is usually advised to pick a meal of the day—such as dinner. Once you eat dinner, you fast for the next 24 hours until you have dinner again the next day. This should ideally be done two times every week, but some people prefer only to do it once every week. It is definitely a tough option, so it is usually not recommended for individuals who are new to intermittent fasting.

The "Warrior" Plan

This is one of the more recent plans that was introduced by Ori Hofmekler, a fitness expert that is well-known in some areas. The plan was introduced to be more of a diet that included intermittent fasting, rather than a special type of scheduled eating plan. It has, however, become very popular among individuals who like to fast, especially those who want to fast due to the weight loss benefits they may achieve.

With the Warrior plan, you get an eating window that only lasts for 4 hours every day. The rest of the day, you will be fasting, but there is a slight twist here. You are allowed to eat unprocessed and whole vegetables and fruits during the day, only a very small amount. At night, you can sit down and have a large meal. As Hofmekler described it, you would "feast at night."

The diet portion of this plan shares many similarities with the popular Paleo diet. In particular, the foods suggested for eating during the day, as well as the foods recommended for your "feast" are mostly based on what you would find in a typical Paleo diet.

Spontaneous Fasting

Finally, we thought it would be appropriate to share some details on spontaneous fasting. This is not a specific type of intermittent fasting plan, diet, or anything of the sort. Instead, this involves those who do not wish to follow one of the plans we have listed above. With spontaneous fasting, you can decide to fast at any given time—there's no need to set up windows. This is done by simply skipping a meal. Do not do this too often—you should know your limits and ensure that you do not restrict your calories too much. You may choose to skip breakfast one day, lunch the next day, and the following day you may decide not to skip any meals at all. Spontaneous fasting is a great way to "dip your toe in the water" and ease yourself into intermittent fasting.

A Note on Liquids

During fasting windows, when you abstain from eating, be sure to drink fluids, especially water. Do not drink anything that has sugar or any calories in it, as that
will increase your insulin and break your fast. Black coffee and unsweetened tea are fine. The occasional

diet soda is not best but can be used initially with the understanding that you are trying to stay away from artificial sweeteners as much as possible—so as you get more comfortable with fasting, you'll later not consume diet sodas.

Getting Started, Step-By-Step

Most people who are used to a daily routine of having three meals and never skipping out will find it intimidating to get started with implementing intermittent fasting into their lives. This especially goes for individuals who eat multiple times a day and who have a particularly hard time controlling their cravings. With intermittent fasting, it is vital that you stick to your schedule for maximum benefits. That said, there is no need to act like you are in a military camp.

With some simple steps, you can make the entire process of adopting intermittent fasting a fun journey for yourself, an experimental procedure that will take some time to perfect, but once you get there, you will be able to master this technique and gain many health benefits. Keep this in mind when you feel like quitting. Remember, you will only be able to reach your weight and health goals if you keep yourself motivated at all times.

Before you jump into intermittent fasting, you might want to take some things into consideration first. In particular, if you have been diagnosed with any type of chronic disease and if you are taking medications, then you should first talk with your physician to determine if this is a safe option for you.

Furthermore, don't overcomplicate things. Start small. Break the process up into small steps. Reach for smaller goals and progress to longer and more difficult fasting windows. If you cave or something goes wrong, do not let it get you down. Instead, just keep on going.

Here is a step-by-step guide to help you out.

1. The first step is to determine what type of technique you want to adopt. The 16/8 is highly recommended for beginners. You can even alter it to a 14/10 technique and then build to the 16/8. What you may not know is that you are already halfway there. You are fasting while you are sleeping. Now, to get to the 16/8, you could skip breakfast, for example or skip dinner.

2. Decide on the time slots—your eating windows and fasting windows. If you follow the 16/8 plan, for example, you can decide to have your first meal of the day at lunchtime, instead of early in the morning, and finish off at 8 PM, for example. Give yourself a good 16 hours without food—this would include your 7 to 9 hours of

sleep, which you should be getting to keep your body healthy.

3. Start small and simple. Try it for one day and see if you can make it. If you feel like you run out of energy too quickly, then stretch your eating window a little and make your fasting window narrower. As the days go by, start to shorten your eating window and make your fasting window longer until you can go without food for 16 hours at a time. If you make a mistake by giving into the temptation of having a snack when the hunger becomes extreme, don't beat yourself up over it. Simply start over.

In addition to deciding on the type of intermittent fast you prefer, it is also a good idea to consider why you want to include intermittent fasting in your life. When you are doing this for a specific purpose, then you will have something to keep you motivated. Perhaps you want to lose weight. This is a great reason to fast. Remember we looked at scientific evidence before that supported the weight loss advantages of intermittent fasting.

If you simply want to help prolong your lifespan and reduce your risk of certain diseases, then these are also important reasons. If you like, write down your reason for fasting on your eating and fasting schedule. This will keep you motivated to ensure you can reach your goal.

Helpful Apps and Tools

Things can become confusing, especially at first when you start with intermittent fasting. This is why using some tools to help you keep track of everything is a good idea. You can always go old school and decide to plot down your schedule on a piece of paper. Perhaps buy a new notebook that is dedicated to intermittent fasting. Write down your schedule and mark down your progress. This will also help you go back and track your performance, as well as see where you have slipped up. Consider slip-ups learning opportunities.

If you prefer to keep things digital, then try out a couple of intermittent fasting apps. You'll surprised at how many there are. Take a look at some—they are available in both the Google Play Store and Apple Store. Consider the user reviews. Then decide on an app that you like and try to use it every day to help you keep track of your journey.

Keto and Intermittent Fasting

The ketogenic diet is the *what* you eat, and intermittent fasting is the *when* you eat. During your eating window, follow the recommendations of the ketogenic diet that we covered in detail in previous chapters. During the fasting window, you abstain from food. During the eating window, you eat according to the ketogenic guidelines.

At the start of this chapter, I told you that the ketogenic diet and intermittent fasting are two very powerful, effective techniques for helping you lose excess weight and maintain your body—down to the cellular level—in an optimum state of health. Now that you've read this chapter and read the many benefits of intermittent fasting, I hope you too are convinced—so convinced that you are going to start intermittent fasting today.

Honestly, intermittent fasting is easy to get started on because there's nothing to buy or prepare. You can do it every day at anytime. It's something that you can start right away by just skipping breakfast—or skipping whatever is your next meal. I recommend to most of my patients that they open the eating period up at noon and eat until 8 PM. Then they fast from 8 PM until noon the next day (eating for 8 hours and fasting for 16 hours). You may think that is hard, but believe me, it will become easy. If you can't go that long, then start at 9 AM and eat until 9 PM (that's 12 hours of fasting and 12 hours of eating). There is no wrong or right way—the point is to start and enjoy the improvements today.

In the next chapter we're going to address an important topic: stalling and setbacks. We'll look at this topic in how it can play out on your journey to reaching your goal weight and also how it can play out after you've reached your goal weight. Of course, I'll be offering great options on how to consider stalls and how to fix any serious stalls. Don't worry—I'm here to help! We can do this!

Randy King's Message

"I tried the 'low carb' before with some weight loss success but never tried the fasting. After trying the fasting for a few weeks, I felt the weight loss was accelerated compared to 'low carb' only."—May 2018

References

http://www.who.int/news-room/fact-sheets/detail/obesity-and-overweight

https://www.niddk.nih.gov/health-information/weight-management/health-risks-overweight

http://becomingeden.com/religious-fasting-traditions/

https://www.healthline.com/nutrition/10-health-benefits-of-intermittent-fasting#section1

https://www.ncbi.nlm.nih.gov/pmc/articles/PMC4414396/k

https://www.ncbi.nlm.nih.gov/pubmed/28715993

https://www.ncbi.nlm.nih.gov/pmc/articles/PMC5674160/

https://www.curejoy.com/content/side-effects-of-intermittent-fasting/

https://www.cell.com/cell-metabolism/fulltext/S1550-4131(17)30612-5

http://www.johnshopkinshealthreview.com/issues/spring-summer-2016/articles/are-there-any-proven-benefits-to-fasting

https://www.ncbi.nlm.nih.gov/pubmed/21527899

Motivation is what gets you started. Habit is what keeps you going.

—Jim Rohn

Chapter 10
Stalling and Keto

As with any weight loss process, you will not lose weight in a perfectly straight downward line. You will have small fluctuations, small ups and downs, and even plateaus at times, but what you want to see is that over time the big picture is a downward trend. This means that over time—even with some ups and plateaus—you end up losing weight.

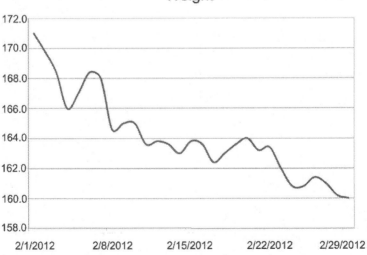

Weight

If you are worried about a few days or up to a 10-day stall, relax. Don't worry about it. Give it time. Losing weight is a marathon, not a sprint. Something else to consider is that you can be losing mass but not weight. What this means is that your waistline and size is decreasing—you are losing inches—but the scales don't indicate, for a period of time, that you are losing weight.

Eleven Options for Tackling a Stall

If you do stall, then do these things in this order:

1 *Track your foods*: you have to know where you are to know where you want to go. Sometimes we are not exactly eating what we think. I have had patients come into my clinic and express frustration that their weight loss stopped after initially losing some weight. What is happening is that after you lose some weight, your body starts to readjust. You may have gone from a diet of 50% to 60% carbs before starting and after you start the ketogenic diet you may end up only decreasing your carb consumption down to 20% to 30%—as you ease your way down to 5% carbs. Because this is a decrease in the carb amount you are used to consuming, initially you'll lose weight. However, over time that weight loss will stall. To get your body into ketosis where the real fat burning happens, you must lower your percentage of daily carbs to 5%. The thing is, if you are not tracking your foods, you won't know if you are really eating 5% of

your total caloric intake in carbs. Think of this like using a roadmap—you have to know where you are at before you figure out where you are going.

2 Increase fat: do this by adding oils, especially olive oil or better yet, MCT oils or real butter. Add an extra 1 to 2 servings per day to your foods. Remember that you can't increase your fat intake by increasing your protein intake. If you think that you can increase your fat intake by eating more hamburger, you will run into problems because in doing that you are also increasing your protein intake. And by increasing your proteins, you may also increase your insulin levels. Remember—insulin equates to fat storage, so you don't want to increase your insulin levels.

3 Avoid the carb creep: if you aren't doing less than 20 grams of carbs per day, then concentrate on achieving this for at least one week. A lot of times, people start off strict, counting every carb. Then as time goes on, they quit counting and start to gradually eat more carbs. While each of us is different and some may be able to increase the carb intake and still lose or maintain weight, if this isn't you and you stall, go back to the basics. Go to 20 grams of carbs per day and see what happens.

4 Decrease protein: if over 20% of your calories come from proteins, then shoot for getting your protein percentage right at 20%. In doing so, you'll be lowering your insulin response. And the lower the insulin, the lower the possibility of fat storage. This is not an all-you-can-eat-meat diet.

5 *Add exercise*: ideally, as you lose weight and start to feel better, your desire to move will increase. This doesn't have to be complicated, especially if you have never exercised in the past or it has been a while. Just start walking, maybe get a Fitbit to track yourself and keep yourself accountable. Then, as a goal, try to add some muscle-building exercises to help increase your metabolism. If you are like most people and you avoid gyms—either because you don't want to go to the gym or you don't have time—do some body weight exercises at home with a small pair of dumbbells. Many different workouts can be accomplished in a small space. Look back at the chapter on exercise for some recommended starter workouts.

6 *Start intermittent fasting*: if you have already started doing some fasting, then add some extended fasts. Remember, fasting is just going without food for a certain amount of time. The easiest way is just to skip breakfast then trying to extend that fast to a longer period of time. By fasting, you re-educate your body on what it means to be satiated versus hungry. As a result, you'll learn to eat only when you are hungry and learn to stop eating once you get satiated. We covered fasting extensively in the previous chapter, so revisit that chapter to decide which type of intermittent fast you want to get started with.

7 Measure your foods: The reason to do this is to ensure you are eating the correct daily ratio of fat, protein, and carbs so that your body stays in ketosis. Measuring my food is something I had to work on. When I ate some loose hamburger in a taco salad, I thought I was eating less meat than I really was. I thought it was 3 ounces, but it was 7 ounces. Another example is the mindless eating of nuts. At night, I found myself eating nuts straight from a bag while sitting on the couch, and I assumed that I was eating a serving. But after measuring the amount, it was more like 3 servings. So without measuring, my intake was much higher than what I was actually consuming. Do I measure everything that I eat now? No, but I did in the beginning, and I do if I start to regain weight or stall. You have to know where you are at if you want to know where you are going.

8 Do a fat fast: a fat fast is a 1-to 3-day plan in which you eat 1,000 to 1,500 calories daily with 80% to 90% of those calories coming from fat: nuts, avocados, cream cheese, etc. If you are keto-adapted, doing this fat fast will accelerate your body into breaking down the fats quicker as all the energy will be from your fat storage. Do not do this for longer than 1 to 3 days because during this fat fast, you will not be getting your vitamins and minerals that your body needs.

9 Check for hidden sugars: you need to get into the habit of reading labels. Sugar can be hidden everywhere, from smoked bacon to almond butter to medications to vegetables. I don't want you to think that following a ketogenic diet is hard, but there is a learning curve to knowing what is in foods. Once you start reading labels you will gain knowledge and get the results that you want.

10 Limit or cut out dairy/nuts: both of these food groups are very high in calories. It is very easy to add many calories without realizing it from eating these. You can eat nuts in large amounts without realizing the calories you are taking in. Dairy can cause a digestive problem for some as well, even though you may not even know it. If you find yourself in a stall, try to cut out both for 1 to 2 weeks and see how you progress. If you see progress, then slowly add these back in and keep track of your goals.

11 Count your calories: take your ideal weight and multiply it by ten. Your ideal weight is the weight you are trying to reach. So if your ideal weight is 200 pounds, then take 200 x 10, which is 2,000 calories. This is the number of total calories per day that you should aim to eat—at the most. If you have stalled in your weight loss, start counting the total number of calories you are consuming per day and make sure it doesn't exceed this number. Also, make sure you are following the fat-protein-and carb ratio prescribed by the ketogenic diet.

Clarification on Fat Adaptation and the Occasional Indulgence

Another area where a stall or setback can occur is around what it means to be "fat adapted." Being "fat adapted" is not the same as being in ketosis. "Fat adapted" means that your body is used to burning fat instead of sugar. When you first start a keto diet, your body has to change and become a fat burner instead of a sugar burner. It takes some time—as we've discussed several times in the book already. To get to being fat adapted, you have to start and stay on a ketogenic diet for a few weeks to months.

You can't start this lifestyle for a few days and expect your body to have totally changed. Most people have a body that for years or decades has used sugar (from glucose from carbs) to get its energy. Starting a ketogenic diet entails changing how the body has spent years fueling itself, and that takes time. The long-term benefit of this lifestyle is that eventually—after you've reached your goal weight—you will be able to enjoy birthday parties, Thanksgiving meals, and the occasional splurge again.

Once you get the results that you want, this is when you can occasionally start adding in foods, like fruits and the occasional ice cream, to your diet. To live the rest of your life without eating an occasional slice of pizza or piece of cake is not realistic. While you are still losing weight to reach your goal weight, you shouldn't add in the occasional indulgence. Later on, after you've reached your goal weight, it is fine on occasion. Yes, eating some ice cream will take your body out of ketosis. However, since your body is now used to burning fat, the switch back to ketosis will be easier—for example, you won't experience the keto flu. Your body seems to be actively searching for the fat to burn, so even if you take in sugars, your body will continue to burn fat. So how does this work, and when and what should you eat?

I followed my plan strictly, eating exactly what I was supposed to eat. I didn't stray and said no to the cookies and pizza. I lost the weight that I wanted, reached my goal weight in only 2 months, and felt better. Since then I have been able to incorporate life—the Thanksgiving meals, the birthdays, etc.—into my ketogenic lifestyle. On my last anniversary weekend, I definitely did not follow a keto plan. I had pizza, pretzels, and ice cream. To my surprise, I actually lost half a pound when I returned. Notice that I only deviated from the ketogenic diet for a special meal, and then I returned to it. As long as the indulgence is occasional, then you will be fine.

One of my patients who had lost 35 pounds on the ketogenic diet was very concerned about gaining weight on a cruise. It was a trip with his wife, and he had been looking forward to it for years. I told him to enjoy himself, and he did. He did gain three pounds, but after restarting the ketogenic lifestyle, his second day in his weight was back exactly where it started prior to his trip. Being able to learn how to cycle in and out of ketosis and teaching your body to be a fat burner is important.

The first step you need to do after you have this plan in place is to reach your goal. Don't deviate and remember your why. Think of this as a savings account for a vacation. If you plan to go to the beach in 12 months, and it will cost $1,200, then you need to save $100 per month. Let's then say you decide to go out to eat and watch a movie, and you spend $100 doing it. Now that money you needed to save is not available and your long-term goal of a beach vacation is going to have to happen one month later. No big deal, you will just go to the beach one month later. But let's say in 2 months you do the same thing and go to eat and catch a movie. Now your vacation is going to be put off another month. The point I'm making is that the more times you deviate from the ketogenic diet—say you eat pie and ice cream—then the longer it will take to reach your weight loss goal. It's best to remember your ultimate goal and work really hard not to deviate, that way you can reach it faster. Once you've reached it, that's when you should consider allowing in more deviations.

After you have reached your goal, this is when you can start adding foods back into your life on occasion. Here again will be different as each of us are different. There are no concrete ways to have one plan for all. The best way that I find that helps my patients is keeping the ketogenic lifestyle on top of mind. What I mean is to continue to track your macros—fat/protein/carbs—on an app and think about what you are doing and what you are planning for. Do you have a trip planned in a week or is Thanksgiving dinner right around the corner? Then use the time before and after to be very strict, eating foods from my keto lists in the correct ratio. Theoretically it would be nice to stay on my plan at all times, but I know that's pretty much impossible (for both my patients and myself), so you have to plan for exceptions—and enjoy them—and then quickly get back into keto.

How often can we go off keto? Again, that's different for each of us. You can use your goals here to help guide yourself. If your main goal is to lose weight, then use your clothes or belt as a barometer. If they start to get tight, then go back to strict keto eating to get yourself back on track. If lowering your sugar was a goal, then continue to monitor those numbers, as they will not lie to you.

Once you have reached those goals and you start to eat things not on recommended and not in the ketogenic lifestyle, it is very easy to let yourself go and find yourself going down a road that you regret. This is why it is so important to keep the ketogenic lifestyle top of mind and not ignore any signs (like very snug-fitting pants!) that you have drifted from your goals.

Weight loss in not a straight downward line as dis-cussed. Nearly all people will experience some setbacks while they are trying to lose weight, not hitting every goal that they have set for themselves. Even after you reach your weight loss goal, there will be times when you will deviate from the ketogenic diet—special occasions like holiday meals and birthdays. Enjoy these deviations, but remember to get back into the ketogenic diet once the occasion has ended.

Whether you are experiencing a setback on your way to reaching your weight loss goal or it happens after you've already reached your ideal weight, remember that setbacks are normal. If you are like me, not everything goes exactly as planned. We have to keep readjusting what we do. Keep these options in mind, referring back to them as you need them. Consult the resources offered on my site as well and check in with other members in the ketogenic community to get their advice on how to deal with a stall or setback: www.ourketogeniclife.com. (Remember to use the discount promo code—BOOK—at www.ourketogeniclife.com/book—that I'm offering exclusively to readers of this book!) This book contains the tools that you need for weight loss and maintaining that weight loss to enjoy a long and healthy life, so keep your goals in front of you, keep going, and you will get results.

Billie R's Statistics

Billie started with a weight of 392 on June 20, 2017. After doing the ketogenic diet for almost a year, she decreased her weight to 347 on May 29, 2018. This is the first time she lost weight and kept it off for so long. Like most, she has had setbacks, but the difference this time is she didn't give up. Her weight remained the same during her times of struggle. She kept tracking her eating, keeping her macros in her mind daily. Billie has struggled with thoughts of feeling like a failure as she has not lost all the weight that she desires. But she has had some success. While she hasn't lost all her weight, she has not regressed to her old habits and has not regained weight.

"If we are growing, we are always going to be out of our comfort zone"

—John Maxwell

Chapter 11
Common Keto Errors

You are learning the ketogenic lifestyle, and with all learning, mistakes can occur. The great thing about mistakes is that they are opportunities for learning. Watch out for these common mistakes, and if you realize you're doing it—then seize the opportunity to learn and change.

1 Too many carbs: this problem is very common, especially at the start. Most people's typical diet consists of an excessive amount of carbs since carbs are in most available foods. Even many vegetables in their raw form contain lots of carbs—think sweet potatoes, pumpkin, and potatoes (all starchy vegetables). If they aren't in the foods naturally, carbs are added during food processing. Because carbs are in so many foods, it can be easy to accidentally consume more than keto's prescribed 20 grams (or 5% of your total caloric intake).

If you follow the list of core keto foods given in chapter 13, then it is very hard to get too many carbs. Too often what I see is that people start eating foods not on the lists. They'll eat things like "diet" protein bars, thinking that because they are labelled "diet," then it must be good for them. In fact, the diet protein bars are filled with carbohydrates. Just look at the nutrition label on the bar to see this! I highly recommend that you stick with the lists found in chapter 13 and don't stray.

If you do stay on the lists and you don't see results, then the next step is to start counting your carbs on an app like MyFitnessPal, an app I use every day. Be honest and diligent, tracking everything that you consume. If are having trouble eating only 20 to 30 grams of carbs per day, then change what you are eating to decrease those grams of carbs.

2 *Too much protein*: protein is important in any lifestyle plan. Protein is made up of amino acids, which are the body's building blocks. There are 20 different amino acids, some essential and some non-essential. An essential amino acid means that the only way we can get that amino acid is to take it in through the food we eat. A non-essential amino acid means that the body can produce it on its own. Out of the 20 amino acids, 8 are essential and 12 are non-essential. So we must eat protein to get those 8 essential amino acids, but the question is: how much protein?

As for proteins, so often we are told we need to eat up to 1 gram of protein for each pound we weigh, especially if we work out. I used to do that very thing. Now it's a lot less. Try to limit your protein intake between 0.6 to 0.7 grams per pound of your body weight. For example, if you weigh 200 pounds, shoot for your protein intake to be (200 x 0.6 to 0.7) 120 to 140 grams.

If you take in more protein than what is called for in the ketogenic diet, then you will halt your progress. The excessive amount of protein will be converted to glucose, which will increase the amount of insulin your body produces. Insulin encourages the body to store fat. Excessive insulin is what we are trying to control. The takeaway: be purposeful in counting your daily protein intake, so you can reach the weight loss goal you've set for yourself.

3 Not enough calories from fat: we have been programmed since our youth to eat less fat. Now, I'm telling you to eat more. It may take several weeks to get your mind around this change, and that is OK. If you are counting calories at the start—don't. Just stay in the recommended ratio of fat/protein/carbs, and listen to your body. Eat when you're hungry; don't eat when you're not hungry.

4 Stress: being stressed is detrimental to your body as it usually manifests through headaches, pains, and stomach problems. It also can produce a chemical called cortisol, which tends to make us resistant to weight loss. I know I can't just tell you not to stress, and then it will all go away, but recognize your stress, realize its potential to damage your goals, and try to take steps to resolve this problem. You may talk with someone, pray, or even visit your medical provider to get help.

5 *Not enough sleep*: as with stress, not sleeping enough can also increase the production of cortisol. To best position yourself to fall asleep easily: don't exercise right before bed, decrease your use of electronic devices in the evening, and don't drink caffeine after 4 PM. If you still have trouble sleeping, consider talking with your provider to get help.

6 *Obsessing over the scales*: so many times I have had patients come in disappointed in what the scales read. They have been following the plan, they feel better, and they have even had to move down a notch on the belt. But they are frustrated with the number on the scale.
I then have to get them to see that changes are happening. The scale is just a snapshot. Don't worry. You are on the right plan to improve your health. A ketogenic lifestyle is a marathon, not a sprint.

7 *Processed foods*: to concentrate on improving your overall health, a goal with the ketogenic lifestyle is to get you eating natural, non-processed foods. Products like protein bars and shakes are not ideal because they are processed (and are likely very high in carbs!). They can be used in a pinch, but don't make them your main foods, especially on a daily basis. And always read the nutrition labels!

8 "It's time to eat" eating: if you are not hungry, don't eat. We all have been trained to eat at certain times that are programmed into our days. Listen to your body as it will tell you when to eat. If you are hungry, eat. If you are not hungry, don't eat. Don't worry about the clock or what your friends and family are doing. Learn to listen to your body.

9 Comparisons: everyone is different and everyone has unique goals. Your progression of weight loss will be different from others as we all lose and gain weight at different rates. It's great to have someone in your corner to encourage you, but don't be tempted to compare your results to their results. The point is to support one another, not to compete.

10 Lack of support: when you're trying to rethink and change what you have been doing for years or decades, you may struggle at times. It's normal. Having an accountability partner will help, keeping you on pace and also encouraging you to continue in your path. At www.ourketogeniclife.com there's a community you can connect with. This is where you can connect with others who are going through the same things that you are going through. It's a way to give support to others, get support from others, celebrate wins, and brainstorm how to overcome hurdles. Engage with the ketogenic community, so you can feel empowered.

Remember, we all will make mistakes. Mistakes are how we learn. The key is when we realize that we made a mistake, we change our behavior.

Though the next chapter isn't the final chapter in the book, it is our conclusion chapter, or wrap-up. We'll revisit the best ways to get started on the ketogenic lifestyle, and then you are good to go to get started. The final chapter offers that fabulous keto food list that so many of my patients rave out. You'll get a list of the core foods you need to easily progress in your keto journey as well as may easy recipes.

Carl S.'s Statistics

Carl was having problems with his liver and eventually was diagnosed with fatty liver. He was sent back to me after finding his A1c was 11.8 on August 29, 2017. After working with me to get on the ketogenic diet and stay on it, his weight went from 244 to 208. But even more impressive: his A1c dropped to 5.8 as recorded on May 23, 2018.

If you fail to plan, you are planning to fail.

—Ben Franklin

Chapter 12
Baby Steps—Progressing to Your Lifelong Lifestyle

Proverbs 16:24 says, "Gracious words are a honeycomb, sweet to the soul and healing to the bones." As you start and progress through these changes in your life, speak encouraging words to yourself. Don't beat yourself up but always keep striving for your goals. Be honest with yourself. If you know what you are doing isn't correct, then find those thoughts and words to encourage yourself to make the right changes. Find an accountability partner who will pick you up as well as keep you on track.

Remember too, you don't have to rush in and do 100% keto and intermittent fasting all at once. If that's your style and it suits you, go for it. However, if that's not how you operate, then ease your way in. Progress little by little.

These baby steps are a review of the most important concepts taught in this book:

1 Start by limiting your carbs to 20 grams a day. As time goes on and you get to where you need to be, then you can adjust your carb intake up or down as needed to keep you where you want to stay.

2 Do not be afraid of fat. This was a big issue for me and most of my patients. We have been told to avoid eating fat at all cost, so switching our mindset on this issue is very difficult in the beginning. Trust the process, it will work. Look to add fat.

3 Remember your why: keep reminding yourself of your goals.

4 Record all three of your macros—your fat, protein, and carbohydrates. This will help you know where you are each day, how you compare to the prescribed ketogenic ratio, and what adjustments you might need in the future. The more that you track your foods, the more mindful you become. The more mindful you become, the more surprised you will be at how it affects your food choices and how it encourages weight loss.

5 Do not overload on protein. Eat what you need, but remember that the ketogenic diet is not an Atkins diet. It's not a high-protein diet.

6 Include intermittent fasting. If not in the beginning, then do so as time goes on. Intermittent fasting teaches you to get in tune with your body, so you can learn to eat when you are hungry, not when the clock says it is time to eat.

7 Remember your fluids and electrolytes—salt, potassium, and magnesium.

8 Do not keep foods at home that tempt you. At the start, you are not stronger than your past urges. This gets better with time, but do not put yourself in a bad situation.

9 Get sleep. This will help your cortisol level.

10 Supplement as needed. Check out the supplement offers at my site www.loveyournewyou.com and enjoy a discount on your first purchase when you put in the code BOOK at checkout.

11 Start exercising. Just start with simple exercises, like walking, and progress as tolerated. In my experience, over 95% of people beginning the ketogenic diet, do not start out doing exercise at the same time. But as the weight comes off, they feel better and more confident. Then they start exercising, which makes them feel even better and more confident. Let this be your experience too!

12 If you stall in your weight loss, go back and review the steps needed to ensure a breakthrough. Remember, if you are 2 or 3 weeks into a ketogenic diet and you haven't seen any weight loss, don't panic. Give your body time to adjust to ketosis. Also, consult with others in the ketogenic community to get advice and support if you experience a stall or at any time in your keto journey: www.ourketogeniclife.com.

Starting the ketogenic lifestyle is a two-fold system. At first, follow the ketogenic recommendations either by slowly adding each step and progressing to add each subsequent step, or jump right in and totally revamp your lifestyle. I have had patients do both ways. The way that's best for you depends on your personality and mindset. Use my website www.ourketogeniclife.com if you want even more information. You'll find there a sample menu plan and recipes to get you going as well as other people enjoying the ketogenic lifestyle that you can exchange ideas with.

Let me leave you with a story that I heard a few years ago: there was a man many years ago who had two fighters whom he trained and entered into boxing contests. Each week he bet on one of the fighters and would always win the bet. Week after week, he would collect his winnings. One day, someone asked him how he would know which fighter would win, never missing out on his prediction. The man responded, "It's simple. I bet on the one that I fed well that week."

From this time forward, what you feed your mind and your body will win out. You have that choice, and you control your destiny. Get started today with a ketogenic diet and with intermittent fasting. Your mindset will change and your body will change. You will be able to live your life and still get the results that you want.

In closing, the next and final chapter offers that fabulous keto food list and easy keto recipes, so you can feed your mind and body keto-style. I want you to reach your goal weight and optimal state of health as quickly and easily as possible—that's where the keto core food list and recipes come in.

Chapter 13
Keto Core Food List and Easy Recipes

What I have learned is that the best way to make changes is to keep it simple. When you read the following plan and types of food, I am purposefully offering something that is easy to do. I have read many articles, books, and cookbooks, and most offer recipes and dishes that are too time-consuming to prepare. Most people who are busy with work and kids just can't or will not do and continue the ketogenic diet if they have to prepare involved dishes. I want to set you up with a plan that I know that you can follow and not overwhelm you—that's the aim of this final chapter.

In my clinic patients come to me seeking ketogenic recipes involving simple foods that are easy to prepare. This is where we start. Getting you to the grocery store and getting the basics is the first steps. After a few weeks, that's when people want to expand and branch out to try new things.

Below is a list of easy and quick meals to get started with, and I'm including some easy recipes afterwards. My patients treasure this list and these recipes. They see it all as their doorway to keto, which is their start to sustained weight loss. Once they reach their weight goals, the ketogenic lifestyle is the one that keeps them on track and healthy. At www.ourketogeniclife.com you'll find more recipes with videos to help walk you through the steps to incorporate different foods that go with the ketogenic diet.

Here's What to Do

To end this book let's return to where I started. When anyone comes to my clinic, saying, "Just tell me what to do," this is where I am going to do just that. With this list of foods and the recipes that follow, I'm telling you what to do to reach your goals and become a new and improved you. Here are simple ways of getting started with different ideas for each meal. If necessary, eat at usual times, but progress to the point where you start to eat only when you are hungry. You'll notice too that no specific amounts of food are recommended. What we are doing is getting you to eat the right kinds of foods.

Breakfast Options

1. Eggs, bacon, avocado

2. Keto coffee: coffee 1 tbsp MCT oil + collagen

3. Crustless quiche: prepare and eat it over a few days, adding full-fat sour cream on it too.

4. Plain full-fat yogurt + walnuts

5. Omelette: eggs, bacon, spinach, and mushrooms, putting full-fat sour cream on top

6. Nothing: this is where most people end up, skipping breakfast and breaking your fast at noon or later.

Lunch Options

1. Leftovers from previous night's dinner

2. Salad with avocado and a protein source. Use a combo of half full-fat dressing and half olive oil. Add bacon to increase taste and fat content.

3. Lettuce-wrapped hamburger. Look to add cheese (not processed) and mayo.

4. Ham rolls with full-fat cream cheese

5. Plate of hard cheese, shaved deli meats, and an avocado and/or olives

Dinner Options

1. Rib-eye steak with salad/vegetables. Use olive oil/full-fat dressing and even melt some butter on the vegetables.

2. Chicken with salad/vegetables. Add full-fat sour cream and olive oil to increase the fat percentages of the meal.

3. Pork chops with mashed cauliflower (recipe to follow)

4. Tuna or chicken salad with a side salad or veggies

Snack Options

1. Pepperoni chips: place pepperoni's on a baking sheet, cover with shredded cheese and bacon bits, and bake at 350 F for 4 minutes.

2. Pork rinds

3. Walnuts

4. Hard-boiled egg

5. 5 Hard cheeses

Core Foods—A Grocery List to Get You Started

Eggs

Olive oil

Avocado

Bacon

Spinach

Yogurt (plain and full-fat)

Walnuts

80/20 Hamburger

Lettuce

Pepperoni

Cauliflower

Rib-eye

Chicken

Pork chops

Shredded Cheese

Bacon bits

Salad Dressing

Cream Cheese (full-fat)

Deli ham

KETOGENIC LOW CARB DIET FOOD PYRAMID

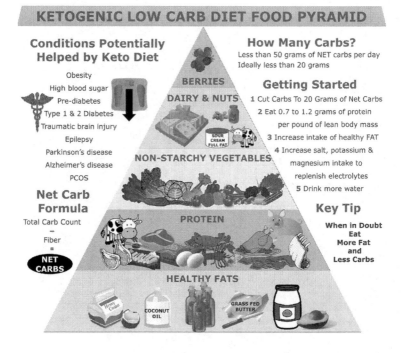

Conditions Potentially Helped by Keto Diet

Obesity
High blood sugar
Pre-diabetes
Type 1 & 2 Diabetes
Traumatic brain injury
Epilepsy
Parkinson's disease
Alzheimer's disease
PCOS

Net Carb Formula

Total Carb Count
−
Fiber
=
NET CARBS

How Many Carbs?

Less than 50 grams of NET carbs per day
Ideally less than 20 grams

Getting Started

1 Cut Carbs To 20 Grams of Net Carbs
2 Eat 0.7 to 1.2 grams of protein
   per pound of lean body mass
3 Increase intake of healthy FAT
4 Increase salt, potassium &
   magnesium intake to
   replenish electrolytes
5 Drink more water

Key Tip

When in Doubt Eat More Fat and Less Carbs

BERRIES

DAIRY & NUTS

SOUR CREAM FULL FAT

NON-STARCHY VEGETABLES

PROTEIN

HEALTHY FATS

COCONUT OIL

GRASS FED BUTTER

Breakfast Recipes

Keto Frittata with Fresh Spinach

Nutrition per Serving: (4 servings)
- Calories 661
- Carbs 4g (2%)
- Fat 59g (81%)
- Protein 27g (16%)

Ingredients:
- bacon (about 150g, diced, alternative—chorizo)
- spinach (225g)
- 8 eggs
- cheese (150g, shredded)
- heavy whipping cream (about 225 ml)
- salt
- pepper

Directions:
1. Preheat the oven to 350 F.
2. Warm some butter on a medium to high heat and fry bacon until crispy.
3. Add in the spinach and mix until it seems withered. When done, set aside the pan.
4. Whisk the cream and eggs together.
5. Pour this batter into a well greased dish.You can use ramekins as well.

6. Add the cooked spinach, bacon, and cheese into the dish, and place it in the preheated oven.
7. Bake it for around half an hour. The dish is serve-ready when the top looks golden-brown and is set perfectly in the middle.

Keto Coconut Porridge

Nutrition per Serving: (1 serving)
- Calories 486
- Proteins 9g (8%)
- Fats 49g (89%)
- Carbs 4g (3%)

Ingredients:
- 1 egg
- 1 oz.coconut oil
- 1 tbsp coconut flour
- 4 tbsp coconut cream
- 1/4 tbsp ground psyllium husk
- A pinch of salt

Directions:
1. Mix all the above mentioned ingredients in a saucepan and cook over medium to low heat.
2. Stir the mixture consistently to create an even texture and serve with coconut cream and fruits.

Low-Carb Blueberry Smoothie

Nutrition per Serving: (2 servings)
- Calories 415
- Protein 4g (4%)
- Fats 43g (87%)
- Carb 10g (9%)

Ingredients:
1/2 cup of blueberries (fresh or frozen)
14 oz. coconut milk
1 tbsp lemon juice
1/2 tsp vanilla extract

Directions:
Add all the ingredients to a blender and blend till you get an even texture. Add to a jar and serve chilled.

Keto Bacon and Eggs Plate

Nutrition per Serving:
- Calories 1,068
- Fat 100g (86%)
- Carbohydrates 8g (3%)
- Protein 27g (10%)

Ingredients:
- 1 oz. arugula lettuce
- 2 tbsp olive oil
- 5 oz. bacon
- 2 tbsp butter, for frying
- 4 eggs
- 2 avocados
- 4 tbsp walnuts
- 1 green bell pepper
- salt and pepper
- 1 tbsp fresh chives, finely chopped (optional)

Directions:
1. Fry the bacon in butter over medium heat until crispy.
2. Remove from pan and keep warm. Leave the fat that's accumulated in the pan. Lower the heat to medium-low and fry the eggs in the same pan.

3. Place bacon, eggs, avocado, nuts, bell pepper, and arugula on a plate.
4. Drizzle the remaining bacon fat on top of the eggs. Season to taste.

Keto Egg Muffin Recipe

Nutrition per Serving: (12 servings)
- Calories 143
- Fat 10g (63%)
- Carbohydrates 4g (11%)
- Protein 10g (28)

Ingredients:
- 8 oz. pork breakfast sausage
- 1 tbsp extra virgin olive oil
- 1/2 sweet onion (thinly sliced)
- 3/4 cup red bell peppers (chopped or thinly sliced)
- 1.5 cups fresh spinach (packed)
- 1 tsp fresh oregano (chopped or 1/2 tsp dry oregano)
- 9 eggs
- ground pepper
- 3/4 tsp salt
- 1/4 cup coconut milk

Directions:
1. Preheat oven to 350 F. Grease a 12-muffin tin.
2. Place the ground sausage in a sauté pan and heat on medium-high. Break up the sausage into crumbles with a spatula as it cooks.

3. When the sausage is half way cooked, add the olive oil, onions, peppers, and oregano to the pan. Saute until the onion is translucent.
4. Add the spinach to the pan and cover with a lid. Cook for 30 seconds, remove the lid, and toss the ingredients. Spinach should be wilted but still bright green. Remove from heat.
5. Place the eggs in a large mixing bowl along with the pepper, salt, and coconut milk. Whisk together until eggs are well beaten.
6. Add the sausage and vegetables to the egg mixture and mix in until well distributed.
7. Divide the mixture between the greased muffin tins (12 total), making sure that each tin has a somewhat equal ratio of eggs/fillings.
8. Bake in preheated oven for 18 to 20 minutes.
9. Cool for a few minutes and remove from tins, loosening the edges first with a knife.

Cream Cheese Keto Pancakes

Nutrition per Serving:
- Calories 365
- Fat 29 g (72%)
- Carb: 8g (9%)
- Protein 17g (19%)

Ingredients:
- 2 oz. cream cheese (organic, will be 1 to 2 carbs per serving, at most)
- 1/2 to 1 packet of Stevia in the Raw (or whatever stevia you like)
- 2 eggs
- 1/2 tsp cinnamon
- 1 tbsp coconut flour

Directions:
1. Blend or beat together all of the ingredients until smooth.
2. You'll make two pancakes, so heat up a nonstick pan or skillet with butter or coconut oil on medium-high heat.
3. Make them just like you would normal pancakes. Try to cook it most of the way on one side and then flip!

4. Top with butter and/or a sugar-free maple syrup (check your labels; they aren't all created equal!).

Crunchy Keto Granola

Nutrition per Serving: (4 servings)
- Calories 562
- Fat 54g (86%)
- Carbs 16g (11%)
- Protein 15g (11%)

Ingredients:
- 1 cup sliced almonds
- 2 tbsp coconut oil, melted
- 1 cup unsweetened coconut flakes
- 1 cup diced walnuts
- 2 tsp cinnamon
- 4 packs Splenda Naturals

Directions:
1. Preheat oven to 375 F.
2. Line a baking sheet with parchment paper.
3. In a medium bowl, toss all ingredients together.
4. Spread out mixture over the baking sheet in as much of a single layer as you can.
5. Place in oven and bake for about 10 minutes or until mixture begins to brown (keep an eye on it; oven times may vary).
6. Remove, mix again, and enjoy in a bowl with cold unsweetened almond milk.

Lemon Blueberry Muffins

Nutrition per Serving: (12 servings)
- Calories 223
- Fat 21g (85%)
- Carbs 5g (8%)
- Protein 5g (8%)

Ingredients:
- 2 cups almond flour
- 1 cup heavy whipping cream
- 2 large eggs
- 1/4 cup of butter (melted)
- 5 drops stevia (or more to taste)
- 1 tsp baking powder
- 1/2 cup fresh blueberries
- 1/2 tsp pure lemon extract
- 1/4 tsp lemon zest

Directions:
1. Preheat oven to 350 F.
2. Zest lemon and melt butter.
3. Crack eggs into a large mixing bowl and whisk until well mixed.
4. Add all other ingredients into the mixing bowl with eggs and mix until well combined.
5. Pour muffins into 12 silicone baking cups.

6. Bake for 25 to 30 minutes (until golden brown and a toothpick comes out clean).

Breakfast Casserole

Nutrition per Serving:
- Calories 354
- Total Fat 26g (66%)
- Carbohydrates 3g (2%)
- Protein 24g (27%)

Ingredients:
- 11 large eggs
- 1/2 cup red bell pepper (chopped)
- 2 cups cauliflower (diced)
- 1 lb. Johnsonville mild sausage
- 1 lb. bacon
- 1 cup sharp cheddar shredded
- 1 tsp salt
- 1 tsp pepper

Directions:
1. Preheat oven to 350 F.
2. Cook bacon and sausage (don't drain) and set aside.
3. Place bell pepper, cauliflower, eggs, salt, and pepper in a bowl and mix well.
4. Pour egg mixture into a 9x13 baking pan and add sausage (mix together).
5. Top with cheddar and bake for 30 to 35 minutes.

6. Remove from oven. Crumble the bacon and add it to the top.

Coffee with Cream

Per Serving:
- Calories 206
- Fat 22g (93%)
- Carbohydrates 2g (3%)
- Protein 2g (4%)

Ingredients:
- 3/4 cup coffee, brewed the way you like it
- 4 tbsp heavy whipping cream

Directions:
1. Make your coffee the way you like it. Pour the cream in a small saucepan and heat gently while stirring until it's frothy.
2. Pour the warm cream in a big cup, add coffee, and stir. Serve straightaway as is, or with a handful of nuts or a piece of cheese.

Lunch Recipes

Bacon-Wrapped Keto Burgers

Nutrition per Serving: (4 servings)
- Calories 896
- Protein 42g (19%)
- Fat 76g (78%)
- Carbohydrates 3g (3%)

Ingredients:
- 7 to 8 oz. bacon
- 20 oz. ground beef
- 3 oz. grilled pickles
- 3 oz. lettuce
- 3 oz. sliced cheddar cheese
- 2 tbsp chili paste
- 2 tbsp cold water
- 1 tbsp olive oil
- 1 tbsp garlic powder
- 1 tsp salt
- 1/2 tsp black pepper powder
- 2 sliced tomatoes
- 1 sliced red onion

Directions:

1. Mix ground beef, water, chopped bacon, spices, and chili paste together. Shape them into burgers.
2. Take bacon slices and wrap them around each burger. Coat each with some olive oil and grill for 5 to 10 minutes.
3. Serve the burgers with a side of tomatoes, onions, pickles, and lettuce.

Keto Tuna Plate

Nutrition per Serving: (2 servings)
- Calories 931
- Carbs 3g (1%)
- Fat 76g (76%)
- Protein 52g (23%)

Ingredients:
- 4 eggs
- 50g baby spinach
- 275g tuna (in olive oil)
- 1 avocado
- 125 ml mayonnaise
- lemon (quarter, optional)
- salt
- pepper

Directions:
1. Start with the cooking of eggs. Place them in boiling water for 4 to 8 minutes. Boil according to your liking, soft-or hard-boiled.
2. Before peeling, put the eggs in an ice bath for a few minutes.
3. Cut the eggs into halves and plate each half alongside avocado, tuna, spinach, a lemon slice (optional), and mayonnaise. Add salt and pepper to taste.

Keto Chicken and Green Beans Plate

Nutrition per Serving:
- Calories 1,009
- Carbohydrates 5g (2%)
- Fat 89g (79%)
- Protein 48g (19%)

Ingredients:
- 7 oz. fresh green beans
- 2 tbsp butter for frying
- 1 lb. rotisserie chicken
- 3 oz. butter for serving
- salt and pepper

Directions:
1. Fry the green beans in butter over medium heat for a couple of minutes. Season with salt and pepper to taste.
2. Put chicken, green beans, and butter on a plate and serve.

Keto Chicken and Feta Cheese Plate

Nutrition per Serving:
- Calories 1,194
- Carbohydrates 9g (3%)
- Fat 102g (76%)
- Protein 62g (21%)

Ingredients:
- 1 lb. rotisserie chicken
- 7 oz. feta cheese
- 2 tomatoes
- 2 oz. lettuce
- 10 black olives
- 1/3 cup olive oil
- salt and pepper

Directions:
1. Slice the tomatoes and put them on a plate, together with chicken, feta cheese, lettuce, and olives.
2. Season with salt and pepper to taste.

Egg Salad

Nutrition per Serving: (4 servings)
- Calories 439
- Fat 41g (86%)
- Carbohydrates 4g (2%)
- Protein 12g (12%)

Ingredients:
- 8 large eggs
- 2 celery stalks
- 2 green onion stalks (tops only)
- 1 green pepper
- 1 tsp yellow mustard
- 2/3 cup mayonnaise
- salt (optional)
- paprika (optional)

Directions:
1. Boil eggs: place eggs in the bottom of a pot and fill with cold water. Bring the water to a rolling boil and turn off the burner. Cover pot with a lid and let them cook for 15 minutes. Remove eggs and place in a bowl of ice water. Allow to cool completely.
2. Chop celery, green onions, and green pepper.
3. Peel and cut boiled eggs, separating yolks from whites. Chop the egg whites.

4. In a bowl, add yolks, mayo, and mustard, and mix well with a spoon.
5. Stir in chopped egg whites, green pepper, celery, and green onion.
6. Top with paprika and salt (to taste). This is optional.

Tuna Salad

Nutrition per Serving:
- Calories 298
- Fat 23g (69%)
- Carbohydrates 3g (4%)
- Protein 21g (28%)

Ingredients:
- 1 can tuna
- 1 large boiled egg (chopped)
- 2 slices bacon
- 1 tbsp chopped onion
- 1 tbsp mayo
- 1 tbsp sour cream
- 2 tsp dijon mustard
- 1/4 tsp dill

Directions:
1. Cook bacon.
2. Chop onion.
3. Boil egg.
4. Open tuna, drain, and place in a small bowl.
5. Add chopped onion and egg.
6. Add all other ingredients and mix well.
7. Top with crumbled bacon.

Chili Cheese Dog Casserole

Per Serving: (10 servings)

- Calories 424
- Fat 34g (72%)
- Carbohydrates 6g (6%)
- Protein 24g (23%)

Ingredients:

- 2 lb. ground beef
- 1/4 tsp black pepper
- 10 hot dogs
- 1/2 tsp ground cumin
- 1/2 yellow onion
- 1 cup low carb tomato sauce
- 2 tbsp low-carb tomato paste
- 4 tsp stevia (optional)
- 2 tbsp worcestershire sauce
- 2 tsp chili powder
- 2 tsp salt (divided)
- 1 cup shredded cheddar cheese

Directions:

1. Preheat oven to 400 F.
2. Brown ground beef over med high heat, and add 1 tsp of salt to meat while cooking.
3. Mix all spices in a small bowl along with tomato sauce and paste.

4. Once ground beef is done, drain and set aside.
5. Add hot dogs to the pan and lightly brown.
6. Remove hot dogs from heat and cut when cooled
7. In a large bowl (or baking dish) mix ground beef, hot dogs, onion, and tomato mixture and mix until well combined.
8. Pour all ingredients into a 9x13 baking dish and top with cheese. Bake for 20 min.

Chicken BLT salad

Nutrition per Serving:
- Calories 837
- Fat 78g (85%)
- Carbohydrates 4g (2%)
- Protein 28g (13%)

Ingredients:
- 1 lb. boneless chicken thighs
- 1 oz. butter
- 1/2 lb. bacon
- 4 oz. cherry tomatoes
- 10 oz. romaine lettuce
- salt and pepper

Garlic Mayonnaise:
- 3/4 cup mayonnaise
- 1/2 tbsp garlic powder

Directions:
1. Mix mayonnaise and garlic powder in a small bowl and set aside.
2. Fry the bacon slices in butter until crispy. Remove and keep warm. Save the grease in the pan.

3. Shred the chicken and season it with salt and pepper. Fry in the same skillet as the bacon until golden brown and thoroughly cooked.
4. Rinse and shred the lettuce; be sure to use a clean cutting board and knife (different from the one used when handling the raw chicken). Place the lettuce on a plate and top with chicken, bacon, tomatoes, and a hearty dollop of garlic mayonnaise.

Low-Carb Onion Rings

Nutrition per Serving:
- Calories 323
- Carbs 5g (7%)
- Fat 26g (74 %)
- Protein 15g (19%)

Ingredients:
- 1 jumbo onion
- 1 egg
- 1 cup almond flour
- 25 tsp grated parmesan cheese
- 1 tsp garlic powder
- 1/2 tbsp chili powder or paprika powder
- 1 pinch salt
- 1 tbsp olive oil

Directions:
1. Preheat the oven to 400 F, or turn on the broiler.
2. Peel the onion and slice into rings.
3. Mix the dry ingredients in a bowl. Whisk the egg in another bowl.
4. Dip the onion rings in the egg batter and then in the flour mix, one at a time.
5. Place the rings on a baking sheet covered with parchment paper.

6. Drizzle or spray oil on the rings and bake in the oven for 15 to 20 minutes. If you are using the broiler, keep a close eye on them; they're done when golden brown and crisp.

Simple Keto Coleslaw

Nutrition per Serving:
- Calories 409
- Fat 42g (94%)
- Carbohydrates 4g (4%)
- Protein 2g (2%)

Ingredients:
- 15 oz. green cabbage
- 1 cup mayonnaise
- 1/2 tsp salt
- 1/4 tsp ground black pepper

Directions:
1. Shred the cabbage with a sharp knife, mandolin slicer, or a food processor.
2. Place in a bowl and add mayonnaise, salt, and pepper. Stir well and let sit for 10 minutes.

Dinner Recipes

Keto Steak and Broccoli Stir-Fry

Nutrition per Serving: (2 servings)
- Calories 875
- Carbs 4g (4 %)
- Fat 75g (77%)
- Protein 40g (18%)

Ingredients:
- butter (about 110g)
- soy sauce (1 tbsp, tamari, optional)
- steaks (350g, ribeye)
- pumpkin seeds (1 tbsp)
- broccoli (250g)
- salt
- onion (1 yellow)
- pepper

Directions:
1. Start with slicing steak, broccoli (including stem), and onion.
2. Warm enough butter in a wok or a frying pan. Fry the meat and season it with salt as well as pepper. Afterwards, remove it and keep it aside.

3. Add some butter to the same pan and fry onion and broccoli till brown.
4. Pour soy sauce in it (optional step).
5. Place the meat back into the pan and stir along with seasoning.
6. Lastly, add in some butter and pumpkin seeds. Serve hot!

Cheddar Mini Meatloaves

Nutrition per Serving: (6 servings)
- Calories 356
- Carbs 2g (2%)
- Fat 26g (66%)
- Protein 32g (34%)

Ingredients:
- 1.5 lbs. (24 oz.) 85/15 grass-fed ground beef
- 1/2 cup yellow onion, diced
- 3 oz. cheddar cheese, cut into 1/2 oz. pieces
- 1 egg
- 3/4 cup ground pork rinds (2 servings, or 18 pieces)
- 1 tbsp butter

Directions:
1. Preheat the oven to 425 F, line a baking sheet with foil, and spray lightly with nonstick spray.
2. Grind pork rinds into breadcrumb-like consistency.
3. Dice onions; sauté in butter over medium heat until caramelized and translucent, and set aside to cool.
4. Season ground beef and add onions and egg; mix thoroughly with hands.

5. Create 6 mini meatloaves and space them evenly on baking sheet.
6. Press each piece of cheddar cheese into the center of each meatloaf.
7. Cover the cheese completely with meat and re-shape the loaves.
8. Cook for 25 minutes or until center is no longer pink.

Taco Bowl

Nutrition per Serving:
- Calories 402
- Carbs 5g (9%)
- Fat 26g (57%)
- Protein 35g (34%)

Ingredients:
- 1.5 lb. ground beef
- 1/2 cup yellow onion, diced
- 1/2 cup yellow bell pepper, diced
- 3 cups fresh baby spinach
- 1 tbsp taco seasoning
- 1/4 cup salsa
- 1 cup shredded cheddar cheese
- salt, pepper to taste

Directions:
1. Preheat the oven to 350 F.
2. Add the ground beef to a skillet over medium-high heat, break into small chunks, and cook until browned and no longer pink.
3. While the beef is cooking, dice the onion and yellow pepper.
4. Add the vegetables to the skillet and cook for 5 minutes until tender.

5. Add the baby spinach and cook for 2 minutes or until wilted.
6. Sprinkle the taco seasoning, salt, and pepper over meat and veggies, and stir until fully combined.
7. Spoon in salsa, stir, then top with shredded cheese.
8. Bake for 15 minutes until cheese is melted.

Buffalo Chicken Pizza

Nutrition per Serving:
- Calories 717
- Fat 54g (67%)
- Protein 48g (26%)
- Carbs 13g (7%)

Ingredients:
- 6 oz.shredded chicken
- 1/4 c medium wing sauce
- 2 cup shredded mozzarella, separated
- 1 cup almond flour
- 3 tbsp cream cheese
- 1 egg
- 1/2 tsp Italian seasoning
- 4 tbsp ranch dressing
- 1 oz. blue cheese crumbles

Directions:
1. In a slow cooker, cook plain chicken breasts on low until tender.
2. Using two forks, shred the chicken into medium-sized pieces.
3. Over medium heat, sauté chicken for about 5 minutes in your favorite wing sauce until all pieces are equally coated and heated through; set aside.

4. Preheat the oven to 425 F.
5. In a bowl, microwave 1 cup shredded mozzarella and cream cheese for about 35 seconds until they start to melt.
6. Add the almond flour, egg, and Italian seasoning; stir together until it forms a dough-like consis-tency.
7. On a baking sheet lined with parchment paper, evenly spread the dough into a rectangle shape. You may want to poke holes in it to prevent air bubbles from forming.
8. Bake the plain dough for 12 minutes until lightly golden brown.
9. Spread ranch dressing on the crust.
10. Top with 6 ounces of shredded buffalo chicken.
11. Sprinkle blue cheese crumbles on top of the chicken; add remaining 1 cup of shredded mozzarella on top of the pizza. Bake an additional 10 minutes until the cheese is melted.

Chicken and Shrimp Stir-Fry with Broccoli

Nutrition per Serving:
- Calories 322
- Fats 17g (59%)
- Protein 31g (32%)
- Carbs 7g (9%)

Ingredients:
- 1 pound chicken, cubed
- 1 pound shrimp, peeled and deveined
- 1 pound broccoli, cut into florets
- 1 small white onion, peeled and sliced
- 3 tsp minced garlic
- 3 tbsp minced ginger
- 1/4 tsp sea salt
- 1/4 cup coconut aminos
- 10 drops liquid stevia
- 2 tbsp coconut oil

Directions:
1. Place a large skillet over medium-high heat, add coconut oil, and when melted, add onions.
2. Let cook for 3 to 5 minutes or until softened, and then stir in garlic and ginger.
3. Continue cooking for 2 minutes or until fragrant.
4. Add broccoli florets and stir-fry for 10 minutes.

5. In the meantime, rinse shrimps and chicken pieces, and pat dry.
6. Into cooked broccoli florets, stir in stevia and coconut aminos, and add chicken and shrimps.
7. Cook for 10 to 15 minutes until chicken is no longer pink and shrimps are cooked through.
8. Serve immediately with cauliflower fried rice.

Keto Fried Salmon with Asparagus

Nutrition per Serving:
- Calories 59
- Carbs 2g (1%)
- Fat 59g (79%)
- Protein 28g (19%)

Ingredients:
- 8 oz. green asparagus
- 3 oz. butter
- 9 oz. salmon, in pieces
- salt and pepper

Directions:
1. Rinse and trim the asparagus.
2. Heat up a hearty dollop of butter in a frying pan where you can fit both the fish and vegetables.
3. Fry the asparagus over medium heat for 3 to 4 minutes. Season with salt and pepper. Gather everything in one half of the frying pan.
4. If necessary, add more butter and fry the pieces of salmon for a couple of minutes on each side. Stir the asparagus every now and then. Lower the heat towards the end.
5. Season the salmon and serve with the remaining butter.

Caramelized-Onion-and-Bacon-Smothered Pork Chops

Nutrition per Serving:
- Calories 691
- Fat 49g (65%)
- Protein 56g (33%)
- Carbs 3g (2%)

Ingredients:
- 4 oz. bacon, chopped
- 1 yellow onion, thinly sliced
- 1/4 tsp salt
- 1/4 tsp pepper
- 4 pork chops
- 1/2 cup chicken broth
- 1/4 cup heavy whipping cream

Directions:
1. In a large skillet, cook bacon over medium heat until crisp. Using a slotted spoon, remove to a bowl and reserve bacon grease.
2. Add onion to bacon grease and season with salt and pepper. Cook, stirring frequently, for 15 to 20 minutes, until onions are soft and golden brown. Add onions to bacon in the bowl.
3. Increase heat to medium-high and sprinkle pork chops with salt and pepper. Add chops to

pan and brown on the first side for 3 minutes. Flip chops and reduce heat to medium, cooking on the second side until internal temperature reaches 135 F, about 7 to 10 more minutes. Remove to a platter and tent with foil.

4. Add broth to pan and scrape up any browned bits. Add cream and simmer until mixture is thickened, 2 or 3 minutes. Return onions and bacon to pan and stir to combine.

5. Top pork chops with onion and bacon mixture, and serve.

Baked Spaghetti

Nutrition per Serving:
- Calories 316
- Fat 20g (57%)
- Carbohydrates 10g (13%)
- Protein 27 (34%)

Ingredients:
- 1 lb. ground beef (cooked and drained)
- 4 cups spaghetti squash (cooked)
- 1 container organic tomato basil pasta sauce
- 1/2 tsp oregano
- 1.5 cups shredded parmesan cheese
- 1 large egg
- cups mozzarella cheese
- 2 garlic cloves
- 1 tsp chili powder

Directions:
1. Preheat the oven to 350 F.
2. Slice spaghetti squash in half and cook in the microwave for 5 to 10 minutes (until you can easily scrape flesh out).
3. After you scrape the insides out, remove seeds and cook for another 5 to 10 minutes.
4. In a bowl combine egg, oregano, chili powder, and garlic. Whisk until well blended.

5. Place ground beef in the bowl and fold in the egg mixture.
6. Roll ground beef into meatballs and cook in a large frying pan for 3 to 5 minutes per side.
7. Place pasta sauce in a small pot and heat.
8. Spray a 9x13 baking pan with coconut oil and coat well.
9. Spread spaghetti squash on the bottom of the pan. Then spread meatballs out evenly on top of it (I make about 20 small meatballs).
10. Cover with parmesan cheese, then heated pasta sauce, and top with mozzarella cheese.
11. Bake for 30 minutes.

Ribeye Steak with Oven-Roasted Vegetables

Nutrition per Serving:
- Calories 796
- Fat 66g (74%)
- Carbohydrates 11g (6%)
- Protein 41g (20%)

Ingredients:
- 1 lb. broccoli
- 1 whole garlic
- 10 oz. cherry tomatoes
- 3 tbsp olive oil
- 1.5 lbs. ribeye steaks
- salt and pepper
- 1 tbsp dried thyme, dried oregano, or dried basil
- anchovy butter (1 oz. anchovies, 5 oz. butter, at room temperature, 1 tbsp lemon juice)
- salt and pepper

Directions:
1. Make the anchovy butter. Finely chop the anchovy fillets and mix them with butter (at room temperature), lemon juice, salt, and pepper. Set aside.
2. Preheat oven to 450 F and make sure meat is out of the fridge in order to get to room

temperature before cooking it. Separate the garlic into cloves but don't peel them. Cut the broccoli into florets. Include stems as well, just peel off any rough parts and slice it.

3. Grease a large roasting pan and place all the vegetables in a single layer. Season and drizzle olive oil on top. Give it a stir to coat and then place the roasting pan in the oven for 15 minutes.

4. Brush the meat with olive oil and season with salt and pepper. Fry quickly on high heat in a frying pan. At this point, you're only looking to give the meat a nice seared surface.

5. Remove the pan from the oven and make room for the meat amongst the vegetables.

6. Lower the heat to 400 F and place the pan back in the oven for a few minutes or up to 10 or 15, depending on how you like your meat—rare, medium, or well-done.

7. Remove from the oven and place a dollop of anchovy butter on each piece of meat. Serve straightaway.

Low-Carb Fish and Chips

Nutrition per Serving:
- Calories 2,034
- Fat 191g (86%)
- Carbohydrates 15g (3%)
- Protein 57g (11%)

Ingredients:

Tartar Sauce:
- 1 cup mayo
- 4 tbsp. dill pickle relish
- 1/2 tbsp curry powder

Chips:
- 1.5 rutabaga
- 1 tbsp. olive oil
- salt and pepper

Fish:
- 1.5 lbs. white fish
- 1 cup almond flour
- 1 tsp salt
- 1 tsp paprika powder
- 2 cups oil for frying
- 2 eggs
- 1/2 tsp onion powder

- 1/4 tsp pepper
- 1 lemon, for serving
- 1 cup grated parmesan cheese

Directions:
1. Mix all the ingredients for the tartar sauce. Place in the fridge while making the rest of the dish.
2. Preheat the oven to 400 F. Peel the rutabaga and cut into thin rods. Brush the rods with oil and place on a baking sheet lined with parchment paper. Sprinkle with salt and pepper.
3. Bake in the oven for about 30 minutes, depending on the thickness of the rods, until golden brown.
4. In the meantime, prepare the fish. Crack the eggs in a bowl and use a fork to combine.
5. On a plate, mix almond flour, parmesan cheese, and seasonings.
6. Cut the fish into bite-sized pieces, approximately 1-x 1-inch, and cover with the flour mix. Dip in beaten eggs and then cover again with flour.
7. Heat the oil in a deep saucepan to 340 to 360 F. (Always keep a lid within reach in case the oil catches fire. Never use water on burning oil. Place the lid on the pan and remove from heat.) You can also use a deep fryer if you have one; follow instructions for your device.

8. Fry the fish for 3 minutes on each side, or until the breading is golden brown and the fish is cooked through. Serve with the baked rutabaga fries and tartar sauce.

Snack Recipes

Spicy Keto Roasted Nuts

Nutrition per Serving: (6 servings)
- Calories 281
- Fat 29g (92%)
- Carbohydrates 2g (3%)
- Proteins 4g (5%)

Ingredients:
- 8 to 10 oz. of almonds, pecans, or walnuts
- 1 tbsp olive oil
- 1 tsp paprika powder
- 1 tsp salt
- 1 tsp ground cumin

Directions:
1. Mix all the ingredients thoroughly.
2. Add these to a frying pan and cook till the nuts are completely warm.
3. Allow it to cool and then serve.
4. For storage, add these to a container with airtight lid and keep at room temperature.

Keto Cheese Puffs

Nutrition per Serving: (3 servings)
- Calories 167
- Carbs 0.2g (1%),
- Fat 14g (75%),
- Proteins 10g (25%)

Ingredients:
- 5 1/3 oz. brie cheese

Directions:
1. Cut the cheese into cubes measuring 1-cmx1-cm. Make sure to remove the rind of the cheese first.
2. Place these cubes onto a parchment paper and place it in the microwave for 1 to 2 minutes.
3. Let them cool and add salt, pepper, paprika powder, or spices of your choice on top.

Keto Chocolate Cake in a Mug

Nutrition per Chocolate Mug Cake:
Calories 405
Fats 37g (82%)
Carbs 6g (6%)
Protein 12g (12%)

Ingredients:
1 large egg
2 tbsp salted butter
2 tbsp almond flour
2 tbsp unsweetened cocoa powder
1.5 tbsp erythritol or Splenda
2 tsp coconut flour
1/4 tsp vanilla extract
1/2 tsp baking powder

Directions:
Melt the butter in the microwave for 25 seconds.
Add the rest of the ingredients and mix well.
If you are making 2 servings, split the batter into 2 ramekins.
Microwave for 60 to 75 seconds.

Chocolate Almond Butter Fat Bombs

Nutrition per Serving: (24 servings)
- Calories 80
- Carbs 2g (1%)
- Fat 9g (98%)
- Protein 1g (1%)

Ingredients:
- 4 tbsp real butter
- 8 tbsp coconut oil
- 4 tbsp unsweetened almond butter
- 4 tbsp unsweetened cocoa powder
- 1 packet stevia or sweetener of choice
- Silicone or plastic mold, 24 cups

Directions:
1. Place butter, coconut oil, and peanut butter in a microwave-safe container, and microwave on high for 35 seconds or until melted; whisk to combine.
2. Add cocoa powder and sweetener, and whisk to combine.
3. Pour evenly into 24 molds. Freeze for at least 30 minutes; store in the freezer in a sealable plastic bag.

Stuffed Mushrooms

Nutrition per Serving:
- Calories 238
- Carbs 8g (12%)
- Fat 18g (66%)
- Protein 14g (23%)

Ingredients:
- 8 oz. baby bella mushrooms, cleaned
- 4 oz. cream cheese, softened
- 1 oz. uncured pepperoni, chopped
- 2 tbsp green onions, diced
- 1 oz. shredded cheddar cheese
- 1 tsp Italian seasoning

Directions:
1. Preheat the oven to 350 F, line a baking sheet with foil, and spray with nonstick spray.
2. Add Italian seasoning, cheddar cheese, diced onions, and chopped pepperoni to the softened cream cheese; stir until thoroughly combined.
3. Clean mushrooms and remove stems; fill each with a generous spoonful of the cream cheese mixture.
4. Bake on the center rack for 15 minutes.

Keto Garlic Bread

Nutrition per Serving: (10 servings)
- Calories 92
- Fat 9g (88%)
- Carbohydrates 1g (3%)
- Protein 2g (9%)

Bread:
- 11/4 cups almond flour
- 5 tbsp ground psyllium husk powder
- 2 tsp baking powder
- 2 tsp cider vinegar or white wine vinegar
- 1 tsp sea salt
- 1 cup boiling water
- 3 egg whites

Garlic Butter:
- 4 oz. butter, at room temperature
- 1 garlic clove, minced
- 2 tbsp fresh parsley, finely chopped
- 1/2 tsp salt

Directions:
1. Preheat the oven to 350 F. Mix the dry ingredients in a bowl.
2. Bring the water to a boil. Add vinegar and egg whites to the bowl of dry ingredients. While

whisking with a hand mixer, add boiling water to mix for about 30 seconds. Don't overmix the dough. The consistency should resemble Play-Doh.

3. Form with moist hands into 10 pieces and roll into hot dog buns. Make sure to leave enough space between them on the baking sheet to double in size.

4. Bake on lower rack in oven for 40 to 50 minutes. They're done when you can hear a hollow sound when tapping the bottom of the bun.

5. Make the garlic butter while the bread is baking. Mix all the ingredients together and put in the fridge.

6. Take the buns out of the oven when they're done and leave to let cool. Take the garlic butter out of the fridge. When the buns are cooled, cut them in halves, using a serrated knife, and spread garlic butter on each half.

7. Turn oven up to 425 F and bake the garlic bread for 10 to 15 minutes, until golden brown.

Keto Oven-Baked Brie Cheese

Nutrition per Serving:
- Calories 344
- Fat 31g (82%)
- Carbs 1g (1%)
- Protein 14g (17%)

Ingredients:
- 9 oz. brie or camembert cheese
- 2 oz. pecans or walnuts
- 1 garlic clove
- 1 tbsp olive oil
- 1 tbsp fresh rosemary, fresh thyme, or fresh parsley

Directions:
1. Preheat the oven to 400 F. Place the cheese on a sheet pan lined with parchment paper or in a small nonstick baking dish.
2. Mince garlic and chop the nuts and herbs coarsely. Mix all three together with the olive oil. Add salt and pepper.
3. Place the nut mixture on the cheese and bake for 10 minutes or until cheese is warm and soft, and nuts are toasted. Serve warm or lukewarm.

Chocolate Mousse

Nutrition per Serving:
- Calories 270
- Fat 25g (85%)
- Carbohydrates 6g (10 %)
- Protein 3g (5%)

Ingredients:
- 11/4 cups heavy whipping cream
- 1/2 tsp vanilla extract
- 2 egg yolks
- 1 pinch salt
- 3 oz. dark chocolate with a minimum of 80% cocoa solids

Directions:
1. Break or chop the chocolate into small pieces. Melt in the microwave (20-second intervals, stirring in between) or using a double boiler. Set aside at room temperature to cool.
2. Whip the cream to soft peaks. Add vanilla towards the end.
3. Mix egg yolks with salt in a separate bowl.
4. Add the melted chocolate to the egg yolks and mix to a smooth batter.

5. Add a couple of spoonfuls of whipped cream to the chocolate mix and stir to loosen it a bit. Add the remaining cream and fold it through.
6. Divide the batter into ramekins or serving glasses of your choice. Place in the fridge and let chill for at least 2 hours.

Bacon Veggie Dip

Nutrition per Serving:
- Calories 233
- Total Fat 18g (70%)
- Carbohydrates 8g (14%)
- Protein 10g (17%)

Ingredients:
- 2 oz.of cream cheese
- 2 slices of bacon
- 2 medium celery stalks (washed and cut)

Directions:
1. Place cream cheese in a bowl.
2. Cook bacon and crumble.
3. While the bacon grease is still hot, carefully pour into the bowl with cream cheese. Add bacon crumbles.
4. Mix well and load celery stalks with dip or simply dip them in the bowl. I found that it is easiest to stuff the celery sticks because you can get all of the grease on the stick.
5. Feel free to use with any other veggies as well!

Snickerdoodle Balls

Nutrition per Serving: (12 servings)
- Calories 121
- Fat 11g (82%)
- Carbohydrates 1g (1%)
- Protein 4g (13%)

Ingredients:
- 4 tbsp butter
- 1 large egg
- 1.5 cups almond flour
- 1/4 cup stevia + 1/8 cup stevia (in a small bowl)
- 6 drops of liquid stevia
- 1/2 tsp vanilla
- 1/2 tsp baking soda
- 1/2 tsp cream of tartar
- 1/4 sp cinnamon (in a small bowl)

Directions:
1. Preheat oven to 350 F.
2. Add 1/8 cup or stevia and 1/4 tsp of cinnamon to a small bowl and set aside.
3. Pour remaining ingredients in a mixing bowl and mix until well combined
4. Remove dough from bowl and shape into 12 balls.
5. Roll balls to coat in cinnamon sugar mixture.

6. Bake for 10 to 15 minutes (check with a toothpick).

To find more keto-friendly recipes and meal plans, please visit www.ourketogeniclife.com. Remember to use the discount code—BOOK that I'm offering exclusively to readers of this book!

Acknowledgments

Writing this book has been harder than I imagined but at the same time has been more rewarding than I thought. I want to thank my editor, Nancy Pile, who helped put my thoughts to paper. Thanks to Scott Allen from Self-Publishing School who guided me through the steps to get here, and also to Debbie Lum, my formatter, who put it all together.

I also want to thank my patients who have helped encourage and motivate me to continue to research and find ways that will give them the best care that I possibly can.

To my family, thank you for your support. The support from my kids—Morgan and David Walker, Zach and Brianna Davis, and Karsen and Justin Cornett—has been felt not just for this book but also in everything else that I do.

Thanks to my wonderful, awesome wife, Dena'. Her support by reading and editing early drafts of this book, to her words of encouragement were instrumental to get this book out to print.

Lastly and THE most important, I want to give thanks to my Lord Jesus Christ. I honestly know that without Him, I could do nothing.

About the Author

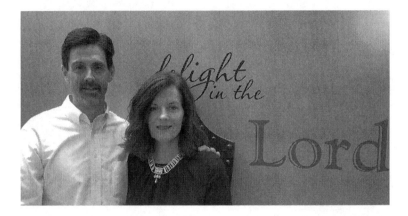

Kevin Davis is a Physician Assistant with over 24 years of experience treating patients, the last 15 years as an owner of his own successful clinic. Because Kevin sees patients of all ages and socioeconomic levels, he is able to relate to nearly everyone's daily struggles.

Kevin is glad to serve in his community, whether as a Deacon at his church or as a volunteer high school basketball coach. He sees giving back as an example of how Jesus came to serve. Kevin was awarded Knott County's Man of the Year Award in 2018.

Kevin and his wife, Dena', are proud parents of three married children and currently have two grandchildren. Since 1994, they have lived in Hindman, Kentucky.

Kevin invites readers to learn more about improving their health with the ketogenic diet and intermittent fasting by visiting the sites www.ourketogeniclife.com and www.loveyournewyou.com.